GIANT CELL ARTERITIS DIET COOKBOOK FOR BEGINNERS 2024

Comprehensive Guide to Polymyalgia Rheumatica and GCA Management – Easy Recipes, Nutritional Plans, and Lifestyle Tips to Reverse Inflammation and Improve Life Quality

Dr. Sarah Matthews

A Heartfelt Note of Gratitude

Dear Reader,

Thank you for taking the time to explore the "Giant Cell Arteritis Diet Cookbook for Beginners: Comprehensive Guide to Polymyalgia Rheumatica and GCA Management – Easy Recipes, Nutritional Plans, and Lifestyle Tips to Reverse Inflammation and Improve Life Quality."

Your commitment to learning about Giant Cell Arteritis (GCA) and Polymyalgia Rheumatica (PMR), and your dedication to improving your health and well-being, is truly commendable. Whether you are newly diagnosed, supporting a loved one, or seeking to enhance your understanding of these conditions, your proactive approach is a significant step toward better health and a more fulfilling life.

Creating this book has been a labor of love, driven by the desire to provide you with practical, actionable, and scientifically backed information to help manage and alleviate the symptoms of GCA and PMR. It is my sincere hope that the recipes, nutritional plans, and lifestyle tips offered here will empower you to take control of your health, reduce inflammation, and enhance your quality of life.

I am deeply grateful for the opportunity to share this journey with you. Your trust in this resource means the world to me, and I am honored to be a part of your path to wellness.

Thank you for your dedication and perseverance. Together, we can overcome the challenges posed by GCA and PMR and achieve a healthier, happier life.

With gratitude,

Dr. Sarah Matthews.

Copyright © 2024 by Dr. Sarah Matthews

All rights reserved.

No part of this book may be reproduced, distributed, or transmitted in any form or by any means, including photocopying, recording, or other electronic or mechanical methods, without the prior written permission of the publisher, except in the case of brief quotations embodied in critical reviews and certain other noncommercial uses permitted by copyright law.

TABLE OF CONTENTS

Introduction

1. Welcome to Your Healing Journey
2. Understanding Giant Cell Arteritis (GCA) and Polymyalgia Rheumatica (PMR)
3. The Importance of Diet in Managing GCA and PMR
4. How to Use This Cookbook

Chapter 1: Understanding GCA and PMR

1. What is Giant Cell Arteritis?
2. What is Polymyalgia Rheumatica?
3. Symptoms and Diagnosis
4. Treatment Options and the Role of Diet

Chapter 2: The Anti-Inflammatory Diet

1. What is an Anti-Inflammatory Diet?
2. Key Nutrients and Their Benefits
3. Foods to Include and Avoid
4. Building a Balanced Anti-Inflammatory Meal

Chapter 3: Kitchen Essentials for GCA Management

1. Stocking Your Pantry
2. Essential Cooking Tools and Equipment
3. Tips for Meal Prep and Planning
4. Grocery Shopping Guide

Chapter 4: Breakfast Recipes

1. Anti-Inflammatory Smoothies and Juices

2. Hearty Whole Grain Breakfasts
3. Protein-Packed Morning Meals
4. Light and Easy Breakfast Options

Chapter 5: Lunch Recipes

1. Nutritious Salads and Bowls
2. Wholesome Sandwiches and Wraps
3. Healing Soups and Stews
4. Easy and Satisfying Midday Meals

Chapter 6: Dinner Recipes

1. Anti-Inflammatory Main Courses
2. Delicious and Healthy Sides
3. One-Pot and Slow Cooker Meals
4. Comfort Food with a Healing Twist

Chapter 7: Snacks and Appetizers

1. Quick and Healthy Snacks
2. Anti-Inflammatory Dips and Spreads
3. Nourishing Small Bites
4. Energy-Boosting Nibbles

Chapter 8: Desserts and Treats

1. Guilt-Free Sweet Treats
2. Fruit-Based Desserts
3. Anti-Inflammatory Baked Goods
4. Simple and Satisfying Desserts

Chapter 9: Meal Plans and Dietary Strategies

1. Weekly Meal Plans for Beginners
2. Customizing Your Diet Plan

3. Tips for Dining Out and Social Eating
4. Monitoring and Adjusting Your Diet

Chapter 10: Lifestyle Tips for Managing GCA and PMR

1. The Role of Exercise and Physical Activity
2. Stress Management and Mindfulness Practices
3. Importance of Sleep and Rest
4. Building a Support System

Chapter 11: Frequently Asked Questions

1. Common Dietary Concerns
2. Adapting Recipes for Special Diets
3. Troubleshooting and Tips for Success

Chapter 12: Resources and Further Reading

1. Recommended Books and Websites
2. Support Groups and Communities
3. Professional Guidance and Consultation

Conclusion

1. Embracing Your Healing Journey
2. Staying Motivated and Committed
3. Looking Ahead: Long-Term Health and Wellness

Glossary of Terms

# Introduction

1. Welcome to Your Healing Journey

Welcome to "Giant Cell Arteritis Diet Cookbook for Beginners." Whether you are newly diagnosed or have been managing Giant Cell Arteritis (GCA) and Polymyalgia Rheumatica (PMR) for some time, this book is designed to be your companion in improving your health through dietary changes. These conditions can be challenging, but with the right nutritional strategies, you can alleviate symptoms, reduce inflammation, and enhance your overall well-being.

This book offers a comprehensive guide to understanding GCA and PMR, along with a wealth of easy-to-follow recipes, meal plans, and lifestyle tips. Our goal is to empower you with the knowledge and tools you need to take control of your health and enjoy a better quality of life.

2. Understanding Giant Cell Arteritis (GCA) and Polymyalgia Rheumatica (PMR)

Giant Cell Arteritis and Polymyalgia Rheumatica are both inflammatory conditions that primarily affect older adults. While they can occur independently, they often coexist, making management complex.

- **Giant Cell Arteritis (GCA)** is a type of vasculitis, which means it causes inflammation of the blood vessels, particularly the arteries in the head and neck. This can lead to severe headaches, scalp tenderness, jaw pain, and visual disturbances. If untreated, GCA can cause serious complications, including blindness.

- **Polymyalgia Rheumatica (PMR)** causes muscle pain and stiffness, especially in the shoulders, neck, and hips. The stiffness is usually worse in the morning and after periods of inactivity. PMR can significantly impact mobility and daily activities.

Both conditions are believed to have autoimmune components, where the immune system mistakenly attacks the body's own tissues. Understanding the interplay between these conditions and inflammation is crucial in developing an effective management plan.

3. The Importance of Diet in Managing GCA and PMR

While medications, particularly corticosteroids, are the cornerstone of treatment for GCA and PMR, diet and lifestyle modifications can play a significant role in managing symptoms and improving overall health. An anti-inflammatory diet can help reduce the need for high doses of medication and mitigate side effects.

The food you eat can influence inflammation levels in your body. By incorporating anti-inflammatory foods and avoiding pro-inflammatory ones, you can support your immune system, reduce pain and stiffness, and improve your energy levels. This book will guide you through the principles of an anti-inflammatory diet, providing practical advice and delicious recipes to help you make informed dietary choices.

4. How to Use This Cookbook

This cookbook is structured to provide you with a clear path to better health:

- **Chapter 1** gives you a deep understanding of GCA and PMR, their symptoms, and the importance of a well-rounded treatment plan.
- **Chapter 2** introduces the anti-inflammatory diet, explaining its principles and benefits, and guiding you on what foods to include and avoid.
- **Chapter 3** focuses on kitchen essentials, from stocking your pantry to essential tools, ensuring you are well-prepared to cook nourishing meals.
- **Chapters 4-8** provide a variety of recipes for every meal and occasion, ensuring you never run out of ideas for delicious and healthful dishes.
- **Chapter 9** offers meal plans and dietary strategies tailored to beginners, helping you incorporate these changes into your daily routine.
- **Chapter 10** discusses lifestyle tips beyond diet, such as exercise, stress management, and sleep, which are crucial for managing GCA and PMR.
- **Chapter 11** answers frequently asked questions and offers troubleshooting tips to help you stay on track.
- **Chapter 12** provides additional resources and further reading for those who wish to delve deeper into the subject.

The recipes are designed to be easy to follow, with ingredients that are accessible and nutritious. Each recipe is crafted to support your health goals, ensuring you get the most benefit from your dietary changes.

CHAPTER 1

UNDERSTANDING GCA AND PMR

What is Giant Cell Arteritis?

Giant Cell Arteritis (GCA) is a form of vasculitis, meaning it causes inflammation of the blood vessels. This condition primarily affects the large and medium-sized arteries, particularly those in the head, which can lead to severe complications if not treated promptly.

- **Symptoms:** GCA can present with a variety of symptoms, including severe headaches, scalp tenderness, jaw pain, vision problems, fever, and fatigue. These symptoms can significantly impact your quality of life, making it essential to recognize and address them early.

- **Complications:** If left untreated, GCA can lead to serious complications such as permanent vision loss, stroke, or aneurysms due to the inflammation and damage to the blood vessels.

- **Causes and Risk Factors:** The exact cause of GCA is unknown, but it is believed to involve a combination of genetic predisposition and environmental factors. It predominantly affects individuals over the age of 50, with women being more commonly affected than men.

2. What is Polymyalgia Rheumatica?

Polymyalgia Rheumatica (PMR) is an inflammatory disorder that affects the muscles and joints. It is closely related to GCA, with many patients experiencing both conditions simultaneously or sequentially.

- **Symptoms:** PMR typically causes muscle pain and stiffness, especially in the shoulders, neck, and hips. The stiffness is often most severe in the morning or after periods of inactivity, and can severely limit mobility and daily activities.

- **Diagnosis:** Diagnosing PMR involves a combination of clinical evaluation, blood tests to check for markers of inflammation (such as ESR and CRP), and response to corticosteroids, which are highly effective in reducing symptoms.

- **Relationship to GCA:** Up to 30% of patients with PMR may develop GCA, and around 50% of patients with GCA also have symptoms of PMR. The overlap between these conditions highlights the importance of comprehensive management.

3. Symptoms and Diagnosis

Recognizing the symptoms of GCA and PMR is crucial for early diagnosis and treatment:

- **GCA Symptoms:** Severe headaches, scalp tenderness, jaw claudication (pain while chewing), visual disturbances (such as blurred vision or double vision), fever, fatigue, and weight loss.

- **PMR Symptoms:** Bilateral aching and morning stiffness in the shoulders, neck, and hips, fatigue, mild fever, and general malaise.

Diagnostic Approaches:

- **Physical Examination:** A thorough clinical evaluation by a healthcare provider is essential. This may include palpation of the temporal arteries, checking for tenderness and swelling.

- **Blood Tests:** Elevated erythrocyte sedimentation rate (ESR) and C-reactive protein (CRP) levels are common in both GCA and PMR, indicating inflammation.

- **Imaging:** Ultrasound or MRI can help visualize inflammation in the arteries and muscles.

- **Biopsy:** A temporal artery biopsy is often performed to confirm the diagnosis of GCA. This involves taking a small sample of the artery for microscopic examination to detect inflammation.

4. Treatment Options and the Role of Diet

The primary treatment for GCA and PMR involves corticosteroids to rapidly reduce inflammation and prevent complications. However, long-term steroid use can lead to significant side effects, making it essential to explore additional management strategies.

Medications:

- **Corticosteroids:** Prednisone is commonly used to control inflammation. The dose is typically high at the start and gradually tapered down to the lowest effective dose.

- **Immunosuppressants:** In some cases, medications like methotrexate or tocilizumab may be used to help reduce steroid dependency.

- **Calcium and Vitamin D:** To counteract the effects of long-term steroid use on bone health, supplements are often recommended.

The Role of Diet:

Dietary changes can significantly impact inflammation levels and overall health. An anti-inflammatory diet can help manage symptoms, reduce the need for high doses of medication, and improve quality of life. This book will guide you through the principles of an anti-inflammatory diet, focusing on nutrient-dense foods that support your health and well-being.

CHAPTER 2

THE ANTI-INFLAMMATORY DIET

1. What is an Anti-Inflammatory Diet?

An anti-inflammatory diet focuses on incorporating foods that reduce inflammation and excluding those that may contribute to it. Chronic inflammation is a key factor in many diseases, including GCA and PMR. The goal of this diet is to support your body's immune response, reduce symptoms, and improve overall health through balanced nutrition.

Key Components of an Anti-Inflammatory Diet:

- **Fruits and Vegetables:** These are rich in vitamins, minerals, fiber, and antioxidants, all of which help combat inflammation. Aim for a variety of colors to ensure a broad range of nutrients.
- **Whole Grains:** Whole grains like brown rice, quinoa, oats, and whole wheat provide essential nutrients and fiber, which can help regulate inflammation.
- **Healthy Fats:** Sources like olive oil, avocados, nuts, and seeds are rich in monounsaturated and polyunsaturated fats, which have anti-inflammatory properties.
- **Lean Proteins:** Include fish, especially fatty fish like salmon and mackerel, which are high in omega-3 fatty acids, as well as poultry and plant-based proteins like beans and lentils.
- **Spices and Herbs:** Many spices and herbs, such as turmeric, ginger, garlic, and cinnamon, have powerful anti-inflammatory effects.

2. Key Nutrients and Their Benefits

Certain nutrients are particularly effective at reducing inflammation and supporting overall health:

- **Omega-3 Fatty Acids:** These are found in fatty fish (like salmon and mackerel), flaxseeds, chia seeds, and walnuts. Omega-3s help to reduce inflammation and can improve symptoms of chronic inflammatory diseases.
- **Antioxidants:** Vitamins A, C, and E, as well as phytonutrients in colorful fruits and vegetables, combat oxidative stress and inflammation.
- **Fiber:** Found in fruits, vegetables, and whole grains, fiber aids in digestion and helps maintain a healthy gut microbiome, which can reduce inflammation.
- **Probiotics:** Found in fermented foods like yogurt, kefir, sauerkraut, and kimchi, probiotics support gut health, which is closely linked to immune function and inflammation.
- **Vitamin D:** Often found in fortified foods and supplements, vitamin D plays a crucial role in immune regulation and can help reduce inflammation.

3. Foods to Include and Avoid

In an anti-inflammatory diet, it's crucial to focus on foods that reduce inflammation while avoiding those that can exacerbate it:

Foods to Include:

- **Fruits:** Berries, apples, oranges, and cherries
- **Vegetables:** Leafy greens (spinach, kale), cruciferous vegetables (broccoli, Brussels sprouts), and root vegetables (sweet potatoes, carrots)

- **Whole Grains:** Brown rice, quinoa, oats, barley, and whole-wheat products
- **Healthy Fats:** Olive oil, avocados, nuts (almonds, walnuts), and seeds (flaxseeds, chia seeds)
- **Lean Proteins:** Fatty fish, skinless poultry, beans, and legumes
- **Spices and Herbs:** Turmeric, ginger, garlic, cinnamon, and rosemary

Foods to Avoid:

- **Processed Foods:** Snacks, frozen meals, and fast food
- **Refined Sugars:** Sugary drinks, candy, pastries, and desserts
- **Trans Fats:** Found in many fried and commercially baked products
- **Excessive Alcohol:** Alcohol can increase inflammation and should be consumed in moderation, if at all
- **Red and Processed Meats:** These can contribute to inflammation and should be limited

4. Building a Balanced Anti-Inflammatory Meal

Creating balanced meals is key to maintaining an anti-inflammatory diet. Here are some tips for building your plate:

Breakfast:

- **Fruit Smoothie:** Blend spinach, berries, a banana, flaxseeds, and almond milk for a nutrient-dense start to your day.
- **Oatmeal:** Top with fresh berries, a drizzle of honey, and a handful of nuts for a satisfying meal.
- **Avocado Toast:** Whole-grain toast topped with mashed avocado, a sprinkle of chia seeds, and a dash of lemon juice.

Lunch:

- **Salad Bowl:** Mixed greens with quinoa, cherry tomatoes, cucumber, chickpeas, and a turmeric-tahini dressing.
- **Grilled Chicken Wrap:** Whole-wheat wrap with grilled chicken, spinach, avocado, and a slice of tomato.
- **Vegetable Soup:** A hearty vegetable and lentil soup, packed with carrots, celery, tomatoes, and kale.

Dinner:

- **Baked Salmon:** Served with a side of roasted sweet potatoes and steamed broccoli.
- **Quinoa Stir-Fry:** Mixed with colorful bell peppers, snap peas, and tofu, seasoned with ginger and garlic.
- **Chicken and Veggie Skewers:** Marinated in olive oil and herbs, served with a side of brown rice.

Snacks:

- **Fresh Fruit:** Apple slices with almond butter or a handful of berries.
- **Nuts and Seeds:** A mix of almonds, walnuts, and pumpkin seeds.
- **Yogurt Parfait:** Greek yogurt with a drizzle of honey, chia seeds, and fresh fruit.

Desserts:

- **Dark Chocolate:** A few squares of dark chocolate (70% cocoa or higher).
- **Fruit Salad:** A mix of your favorite fruits, topped with a dollop of yogurt.

- **Baked Apples:** Stuffed with nuts and a sprinkle of cinnamon, baked until tender.

By following these guidelines, you can create meals that are both delicious and beneficial for managing GCA and PMR.

CHAPTER 3

KITCHEN ESSENTIALS

1. Stocking Your Pantry

Creating an anti-inflammatory diet starts with having the right ingredients on hand. Here's a comprehensive list of pantry staples to ensure you're always prepared to make healthy, anti-inflammatory meals.

Grains and Legumes:

- **Quinoa:** High in protein and fiber, quinoa is a versatile base for many dishes.//
- **Brown Rice:** A whole grain that provides steady energy and essential nutrients.
- **Oats:** Ideal for breakfast and baking, rich in fiber and nutrients.
- **Lentils and Beans:** Excellent plant-based protein sources that are also high in fiber.
- **Whole-Wheat Pasta:** A healthier alternative to refined pasta.

Healthy Fats:

- **Extra Virgin Olive Oil:** A primary source of monounsaturated fats and antioxidants.
- **Coconut Oil:** Good for cooking at higher temperatures.
- **Avocado Oil:** Another excellent cooking oil with a high smoke point.

- **Nuts and Seeds:** Almonds, walnuts, chia seeds, flaxseeds, and pumpkin seeds.

Proteins:

- **Canned Fish:** Such as salmon and sardines, which are high in omega-3 fatty acids.

- **Dried or Canned Beans:** Including black beans, chickpeas, and lentils.

- **Nuts and Nut Butters:** Almond butter and peanut butter, without added sugars or oils.

- **Tofu and Tempeh:** Great plant-based protein options.

Spices and Herbs:

- **Turmeric:** Known for its powerful anti-inflammatory properties.

- **Ginger:** Adds flavor and has anti-inflammatory benefits.

- **Garlic:** An essential ingredient with numerous health benefits.

- **Cinnamon:** Can help regulate blood sugar and reduce inflammation.

- **Dried Herbs:** Such as oregano, thyme, basil, and rosemary.

Fruits and Vegetables:

- **Canned Tomatoes:** For sauces, soups, and stews.

- **Dried Fruits:** Such as apricots, raisins, and cranberries (without added sugar).

- **Frozen Vegetables:** Such as spinach, peas, and mixed vegetables for quick meals.

- **Frozen Berries:** High in antioxidants and perfect for smoothies and desserts.

Miscellaneous:

- **Low-Sodium Broth:** Chicken, beef, or vegetable broth for soups and cooking grains.

- **Apple Cider Vinegar:** Great for dressings and marinades.

- **Honey or Maple Syrup:** Natural sweeteners for baking and cooking.

- **Dark Chocolate:** For a healthy treat, choose 70% cocoa or higher.

2. Essential Kitchen Tools

Having the right tools can make cooking more enjoyable and efficient. Here's a list of essential kitchen tools for preparing anti-inflammatory meals:

Cookware:

- **Nonstick Skillet:** Ideal for sautéing vegetables and proteins with minimal oil.

- **Large Pot:** For soups, stews, and cooking grains.

- **Baking Sheets:** For roasting vegetables and baking healthy treats.

- **Slow Cooker:** For making easy, set-it-and-forget-it meals.

- **Blender:** For smoothies, soups, and sauces.

- **Food Processor:** Useful for chopping, mixing, and creating healthy dips and spreads.

Utensils:

- **Sharp Knives:** A chef's knife and paring knife for chopping and slicing.
- **Cutting Boards:** At least one for vegetables and another for proteins.
- **Mixing Bowls:** Various sizes for prepping ingredients.
- **Measuring Cups and Spoons:** For accurate measurements.
- **Wooden Spoons and Spatulas:** Gentle on cookware and versatile.
- **Vegetable Peeler:** For peeling fruits and vegetables.
- **Whisk:** For mixing dressings and batters.
- **Colander:** For draining pasta and rinsing vegetables and legumes.

Appliances:

- **Electric Mixer:** For baking and mixing ingredients.
- **Toaster Oven:** For quick and convenient cooking.
- **Instant Pot:** A versatile appliance for pressure cooking, slow cooking, and more.

3. Tips for Meal Planning and Preparation

Planning and preparing meals in advance can help you stay on track with your anti-inflammatory diet. Here are some tips to make meal planning and preparation easier:

Plan Your Meals:

- **Weekly Planning:** Spend some time each week planning your meals. Consider what recipes you want to try and create a shopping list.

- **Balanced Meals:** Ensure each meal includes a source of protein, healthy fat, whole grains, and plenty of vegetables.

- **Batch Cooking:** Cook larger portions of meals that can be easily reheated, such as soups, stews, and casseroles.

Prepping Ingredients:

- **Chop Vegetables Ahead of Time:** Wash and chop vegetables for the week to save time during busy days.

- **Cook Grains in Advance:** Prepare a batch of quinoa, brown rice, or oats to have on hand for quick meals.

- **Portion Snacks:** Pre-portion nuts, fruits, and other snacks to avoid unhealthy choices.

Storage Tips:

- **Use Glass Containers:** Store prepped ingredients and meals in airtight glass containers to keep them fresh.

- **Label and Date:** Label containers with the contents and date to keep track of freshness.

- **Freeze Portions:** Freeze portions of meals for later use, especially when you make large batches.

Cooking Strategies:

- **One-Pot Meals:** Simplify cleanup by making one-pot meals that combine proteins, grains, and vegetables.

- **Sheet Pan Dinners:** Roast proteins and vegetables together on a baking sheet for an easy and nutritious meal.
- **Use a Slow Cooker or Instant Pot:** These appliances can save time and effort, especially for soups, stews, and braised dishes.

By stocking your pantry with healthy staples, equipping your kitchen with essential tools, and using effective meal planning and preparation strategies, you can make cooking and eating anti-inflammatory meals a seamless and enjoyable part of your routine.

4. Grocery Shopping Guide

Navigating the grocery store with an anti-inflammatory diet in mind can be straightforward when you know what to look for. This guide will help you make informed choices, ensuring you have everything you need for a healthy, anti-inflammatory diet.

General Tips for Grocery Shopping:

- **Shop the Perimeter:** Fresh produce, meats, dairy, and whole grains are often found around the store's perimeter. Processed and packaged foods, which are generally less healthy, tend to be in the center aisles.
- **Read Labels:** Look for items with minimal ingredients and no added sugars, artificial preservatives, or unhealthy fats. Ingredients should be recognizable and whole foods.
- **Choose Fresh and Whole Foods:** Whenever possible, opt for fresh, whole foods over processed options. These are typically more nutrient-dense and free from additives.

- **Buy Organic When Possible:** Organic produce can reduce your exposure to pesticides. If budget is a concern, prioritize buying organic for the "Dirty Dozen" list of produce with the highest pesticide residues.

- **Plan Ahead:** Make a list based on your meal plan to avoid impulse purchases and ensure you have all the ingredients you need for your recipes.

Produce:

- **Fruits:** Apples, berries (blueberries, strawberries, raspberries), oranges, pears, grapes, bananas, and citrus fruits. Fresh and frozen options are both good choices.

- **Vegetables:** Leafy greens (spinach, kale, Swiss chard), cruciferous vegetables (broccoli, cauliflower, Brussels sprouts), root vegetables (sweet potatoes, carrots, beets), and other veggies (bell peppers, zucchini, cucumbers, tomatoes).

- **Herbs:** Fresh herbs like parsley, cilantro, basil, thyme, and rosemary can enhance flavor and offer health benefits.

Grains and Legumes:

- **Whole Grains:** Brown rice, quinoa, barley, farro, bulgur, whole-wheat pasta, and oats.

- **Legumes:** Dried or canned beans (black beans, chickpeas, kidney beans, lentils).

Proteins:

- **Fish:** Fresh or frozen salmon, mackerel, sardines, and other fatty fish rich in omega-3s.

- **Poultry:** Organic or free-range chicken and turkey.

- **Tofu and Tempeh:** Non-GMO and organic options if possible.
- **Eggs:** Free-range or organic eggs.

Dairy and Alternatives:

- **Yogurt:** Greek yogurt or other high-protein options, preferably unsweetened and with live cultures.
- **Milk Alternatives:** Almond milk, coconut milk, oat milk, and other plant-based options without added sugars.
- **Cheese:** Moderation is key; choose natural, minimally processed cheeses.

Nuts, Seeds, and Oils:

- **Nuts:** Almonds, walnuts, pecans, and pistachios. Opt for raw or dry-roasted without added oils or salts.
- **Seeds:** Chia seeds, flaxseeds, pumpkin seeds, and sunflower seeds.
- **Oils:** Extra virgin olive oil, coconut oil, avocado oil.

Spices and Condiments:

- **Spices:** Turmeric, ginger, cinnamon, cumin, coriander, paprika, and black pepper.
- **Condiments:** Mustard, apple cider vinegar, balsamic vinegar, and low-sodium soy sauce or tamari.
- **Herbs:** Fresh or dried options like oregano, thyme, rosemary, and basil.

Beverages:

- **Water:** Essential for hydration. Consider adding lemon or cucumber slices for flavor.

- **Herbal Teas:** Green tea, chamomile, and other caffeine-free options.

- **Smoothie Ingredients:** Unsweetened almond milk, coconut water, and various frozen fruits and vegetables.

Snacks:

- **Fruits and Vegetables:** Pre-cut veggies like carrot sticks, cucumber slices, and apple wedges.

- **Healthy Snack Bars:** Look for bars with whole food ingredients and minimal added sugar.

- **Hummus and Guacamole:** Perfect for dipping vegetables or spreading on whole-grain crackers.

Grocery Shopping Tips:

- **Seasonal and Local Produce:** Opt for seasonal fruits and vegetables to ensure freshness and better prices. Local farmers' markets are excellent sources of fresh produce.

- **Bulk Buying:** Consider buying grains, nuts, and seeds in bulk to save money and reduce packaging waste.

- **Sales and Coupons:** Take advantage of sales and use coupons for healthy items to manage your grocery budget.

By following this guide, you can ensure your kitchen is always stocked with the essentials for preparing delicious and nutritious anti-inflammatory meals. With the right ingredients on hand, maintaining your diet will be easier and more enjoyable.

CHAPTER 4

BREAKFAST RECIPES

Breakfast is the most important meal of the day, especially when managing conditions like Giant Cell Arteritis (GCA) and Polymyalgia Rheumatica (PMR). Starting your day with anti-inflammatory foods can help reduce symptoms and provide sustained energy. Here are some detailed, delicious, and nutrient-rich breakfast recipes designed to combat inflammation.

1. Anti-Inflammatory Smoothie Bowl

Ingredients:

- 1 cup frozen mixed berries (blueberries, strawberries, raspberries)
- 1 banana, sliced
- 1 cup unsweetened almond milk or coconut milk
- 1 tablespoon chia seeds
- 1 tablespoon flaxseeds
- 1 teaspoon turmeric powder
- 1 teaspoon honey or maple syrup (optional)
- Toppings: fresh berries, sliced banana, granola, coconut flakes, and almond butter

Instructions:

1. In a blender, combine the frozen berries, banana, almond milk, chia seeds, flaxseeds, turmeric powder, and honey or maple syrup (if using). Blend until smooth.

2. Pour the smoothie into a bowl.
3. Top with fresh berries, sliced banana, granola, coconut flakes, and a drizzle of almond butter.
4. Enjoy immediately for a refreshing and nutrient-packed start to your day.

Benefits: This smoothie bowl is rich in antioxidants, fiber, and healthy fats. Turmeric adds powerful anti-inflammatory properties, while the berries provide a high dose of vitamins and antioxidants.

---

2. Quinoa Breakfast Porridge

Ingredients:

- 1 cup cooked quinoa
- 1 cup unsweetened almond milk
- 1 tablespoon chia seeds
- 1 tablespoon almond butter
- 1 tablespoon maple syrup
- 1 teaspoon vanilla extract
- 1/2 teaspoon ground cinnamon
- Toppings: fresh berries, sliced banana, chopped nuts, and a drizzle of honey

Instructions:

1. In a medium saucepan, combine the cooked quinoa and almond milk. Bring to a simmer over medium heat.
2. Stir in the chia seeds, almond butter, maple syrup, vanilla extract, and ground cinnamon.

3. Cook, stirring occasionally, until the mixture thickens and is heated through, about 5-7 minutes.
4. Serve the porridge in bowls and top with fresh berries, sliced banana, chopped nuts, and a drizzle of honey.
5. Enjoy warm.

Benefits: Quinoa is a complete protein, providing all nine essential amino acids. This porridge is also high in fiber, healthy fats, and antioxidants, making it an excellent choice for a filling and anti-inflammatory breakfast.

---

3. Avocado and Egg Toast

Ingredients:

- 1 ripe avocado
- 2 slices of whole-grain or sourdough bread
- 2 large eggs
- 1 tablespoon olive oil
- Salt and pepper to taste
- Red pepper flakes (optional)
- Fresh herbs (optional: cilantro, parsley, or chives)

Instructions:

1. Toast the bread slices to your desired level of crispiness.
2. While the bread is toasting, heat the olive oil in a small skillet over medium heat. Crack the eggs into the skillet and cook until the whites are set but the yolks are still runny, about 3-4 minutes.

3. While the eggs are cooking, mash the avocado in a bowl and season with salt and pepper.
4. Spread the mashed avocado evenly over the toasted bread slices.
5. Top each slice with a fried egg. Sprinkle with red pepper flakes and fresh herbs, if using.
6. Serve immediately.

Benefits: Avocado provides healthy monounsaturated fats and a variety of vitamins and minerals. Eggs are a great source of protein and essential nutrients. Together, they make a balanced, anti-inflammatory breakfast that is both satisfying and delicious.

---

4. Turmeric-Spiced Oatmeal

Ingredients:

- 1 cup rolled oats
- 2 cups unsweetened almond milk or water
- 1 teaspoon ground turmeric
- 1/2 teaspoon ground cinnamon
- 1 tablespoon maple syrup or honey
- 1/4 teaspoon black pepper (to enhance the absorption of turmeric)
- Toppings: sliced banana, blueberries, chopped nuts, and a drizzle of almond butter

Instructions:

1. In a medium saucepan, bring the almond milk or water to a boil.

2. Stir in the rolled oats, ground turmeric, ground cinnamon, and black pepper.
3. Reduce the heat to medium-low and cook, stirring occasionally, until the oats are tender and the mixture has thickened, about 5 minutes.
4. Remove from heat and stir in the maple syrup or honey.
5. Serve the oatmeal in bowls and top with sliced banana, blueberries, chopped nuts, and a drizzle of almond butter.
6. Enjoy warm.

Benefits: This oatmeal is packed with anti-inflammatory spices like turmeric and cinnamon, which not only add flavor but also provide significant health benefits. The combination of oats and toppings offers a balanced mix of fiber, protein, and healthy fats.

---

5. Chia Seed Pudding

Ingredients:

- 1/4 cup chia seeds
- 1 cup unsweetened almond milk
- 1 tablespoon maple syrup or honey
- 1/2 teaspoon vanilla extract
- Toppings: fresh berries, sliced banana, granola, and a sprinkle of cinnamon

Instructions:

1. In a bowl or jar, combine the chia seeds, almond milk, maple syrup or honey, and vanilla extract. Stir well to mix.

2. Cover and refrigerate for at least 4 hours, or overnight, until the chia seeds have absorbed the liquid and the mixture has thickened to a pudding-like consistency.
3. Before serving, stir the pudding to ensure an even texture.
4. Divide the pudding into bowls and top with fresh berries, sliced banana, granola, and a sprinkle of cinnamon.
5. Enjoy cold.

Benefits: Chia seeds are a powerhouse of nutrition, providing omega-3 fatty acids, fiber, and protein. This pudding is easy to prepare ahead of time and makes a convenient and nutrient-dense breakfast option.

---

6. Green Smoothie

Ingredients:

- 1 cup spinach or kale leaves, packed
- 1 banana
- 1/2 avocado
- 1 cup unsweetened almond milk
- 1 tablespoon chia seeds
- 1 tablespoon flaxseeds
- 1 teaspoon honey or maple syrup (optional)
- 1/2 teaspoon ground ginger (optional)

Instructions:

1. In a blender, combine the spinach or kale, banana, avocado, almond milk, chia seeds, flaxseeds, honey or maple syrup (if using), and ground ginger (if using).

2. Blend until smooth and creamy.
3. Pour into a glass and serve immediately.

Benefits: This green smoothie is packed with leafy greens, healthy fats, and fiber. It's a refreshing and energizing way to start your day, providing a host of anti-inflammatory nutrients.

With these detailed breakfast recipes, you'll have a variety of delicious and nutritious options to start your day on the right foot. Each recipe is designed to support your anti-inflammatory diet and provide the energy you need to manage GCA and PMR effectively.

2. Hearty Whole Grain Breakfasts

a. Steel-Cut Oats with Berries and Nuts

Ingredients:

- 1 cup steel-cut oats
- 4 cups water or unsweetened almond milk
- 1 cup mixed berries (blueberries, strawberries, raspberries)
- 1/4 cup chopped nuts (walnuts, almonds, pecans)
- 1 tablespoon chia seeds
- 1 teaspoon ground cinnamon
- 1 tablespoon honey or maple syrup (optional)

Instructions:

1. In a medium saucepan, bring the water or almond milk to a boil.
2. Stir in the steel-cut oats, reduce the heat to low, and simmer uncovered, stirring occasionally, for about 20-30 minutes, or until the oats reach your desired consistency.
3. Remove from heat and let the oats sit for a few minutes to thicken.
4. Divide the oats into bowls and top with mixed berries, chopped nuts, chia seeds, and a sprinkle of ground cinnamon.
5. Drizzle with honey or maple syrup if desired.
6. Serve warm.

Benefits: Steel-cut oats are less processed than rolled oats, offering more fiber and a lower glycemic index, which helps stabilize blood sugar levels. Topping with berries and nuts adds antioxidants, healthy fats, and additional fiber.

b. Quinoa and Fruit Breakfast Bowl

Ingredients:

- 1 cup cooked quinoa
- 1/2 cup unsweetened almond milk
- 1/2 teaspoon vanilla extract
- 1 tablespoon maple syrup or honey
- 1/2 cup fresh fruit (sliced bananas, strawberries, blueberries)
- 1 tablespoon chopped nuts (almonds, walnuts)
- 1 tablespoon chia seeds

Instructions:

1. In a medium saucepan, combine the cooked quinoa, almond milk, vanilla extract, and maple syrup or honey.
2. Cook over medium heat until warmed through, about 3-5 minutes.
3. Divide the quinoa mixture into bowls.
4. Top with fresh fruit, chopped nuts, and chia seeds.
5. Serve immediately.

Benefits: Quinoa is a complete protein and provides essential amino acids. This breakfast bowl combines protein, fiber, and healthy fats to keep you full and energized.

3. Protein-Packed Morning Meals

a. Veggie-Packed Omelet

Ingredients:

- 3 large eggs (or egg whites for a lighter option)
- 1/4 cup chopped spinach
- 1/4 cup chopped bell peppers (red, yellow, or green)
- 1/4 cup chopped mushrooms
- 1/4 cup diced tomatoes
- 1/4 cup feta cheese (optional)
- 1 tablespoon olive oil
- Salt and pepper to taste
- Fresh herbs (optional: parsley, cilantro)

Instructions:

1. In a medium bowl, whisk the eggs and season with salt and pepper.
2. Heat the olive oil in a nonstick skillet over medium heat.
3. Add the chopped vegetables and sauté until tender, about 3-5 minutes.
4. Pour the eggs over the vegetables and cook until the edges begin to set.
5. Sprinkle with feta cheese, if using.
6. Carefully fold the omelet in half and cook until fully set.
7. Garnish with fresh herbs and serve immediately.

Benefits: This omelet is packed with protein and vegetables, providing essential vitamins and minerals. Eggs are a great source of high-quality protein, and the veggies add fiber and antioxidants.

b. Greek Yogurt Parfait

Ingredients:

- 1 cup Greek yogurt (plain, unsweetened)
- 1/2 cup fresh or frozen berries (blueberries, raspberries, strawberries)
- 1/4 cup granola (choose a low-sugar option)
- 1 tablespoon honey or maple syrup
- 1 tablespoon chia seeds

Instructions:

1. In a glass or bowl, layer the Greek yogurt, berries, granola, and chia seeds.
2. Drizzle with honey or maple syrup.
3. Repeat the layers if desired for a taller parfait.
4. Serve immediately.

Benefits: Greek yogurt is high in protein and probiotics, which support gut health. Berries add antioxidants, while granola and chia seeds provide fiber and healthy fats.

4. Light and Easy Breakfast Options

a. Avocado and Tomato Toast

Ingredients:

- 1 ripe avocado
- 2 slices whole-grain bread
- 1 medium tomato, sliced
- Salt and pepper to taste
- Red pepper flakes (optional)
- Fresh basil or cilantro (optional)

Instructions:

1. Toast the whole-grain bread to your desired level of crispiness.
2. While the bread is toasting, mash the avocado in a small bowl and season with salt and pepper.
3. Spread the mashed avocado evenly over the toasted bread slices.
4. Top with sliced tomato.
5. Sprinkle with red pepper flakes and fresh herbs if desired.
6. Serve immediately.

Benefits: This simple yet nutritious breakfast provides healthy fats from the avocado, whole grains from the bread, and antioxidants from the tomatoes. It's quick to prepare and satisfying.

b. Chia Seed Pudding

Ingredients:

- 1/4 cup chia seeds
- 1 cup unsweetened almond milk
- 1 tablespoon maple syrup or honey
- 1/2 teaspoon vanilla extract
- Toppings: fresh berries, sliced banana, granola, and a sprinkle of cinnamon

Instructions:

1. In a bowl or jar, combine the chia seeds, almond milk, maple syrup or honey, and vanilla extract. Stir well to mix.
2. Cover and refrigerate for at least 4 hours, or overnight, until the chia seeds have absorbed the liquid and the mixture has thickened to a pudding-like consistency.
3. Before serving, stir the pudding to ensure an even texture.
4. Divide the pudding into bowls and top with fresh berries, sliced banana, granola, and a sprinkle of cinnamon.
5. Enjoy cold.

Benefits: Chia seeds are a powerhouse of nutrition, providing omega-3 fatty acids, fiber, and protein. This pudding is easy to prepare ahead of time and makes a convenient and nutrient-dense breakfast option.

c. Green Smoothie

Ingredients:

- 1 cup spinach or kale leaves, packed
- 1 banana
- 1/2 avocado
- 1 cup unsweetened almond milk
- 1 tablespoon chia seeds
- 1 tablespoon flaxseeds
- 1 teaspoon honey or maple syrup (optional)
- 1/2 teaspoon ground ginger (optional)

Instructions:

1. In a blender, combine the spinach or kale, banana, avocado, almond milk, chia seeds, flaxseeds, honey or maple syrup (if using), and ground ginger (if using).
2. Blend until smooth and creamy.
3. Pour into a glass and serve immediately.

Benefits: This green smoothie is packed with leafy greens, healthy fats, and fiber. It's a refreshing and energizing way to start your day, providing a host of anti-inflammatory nutrients.

With these additional sections, you now have a complete and detailed guide to a variety of anti-inflammatory breakfast options. Each recipe is designed to support your health and help manage GCA and PMR effectively.

CHAPTER 5

LUNCH RECIPES

Lunch is an important meal that helps sustain energy and provide essential nutrients to keep you going through the day. For individuals managing Giant Cell Arteritis (GCA) and Polymyalgia Rheumatica (PMR), it's crucial to focus on anti-inflammatory foods that promote healing and overall well-being. Here are some detailed and delicious lunch recipes tailored to these needs.

1. Nutritious Salads and Bowls

a. Quinoa and Kale Salad with Lemon-Tahini Dressing

Ingredients:

- 1 cup cooked quinoa
- 2 cups kale, finely chopped
- 1/2 cup cherry tomatoes, halved
- 1/2 cucumber, diced
- 1/4 cup red onion, thinly sliced
- 1/4 cup toasted pumpkin seeds
- 1/4 cup crumbled feta cheese (optional)

Lemon-Tahini Dressing:

- 1/4 cup tahini
- 1/4 cup fresh lemon juice

- 1 tablespoon olive oil
- 1 tablespoon maple syrup or honey
- 1 clove garlic, minced
- Salt and pepper to taste
- Water to thin, if necessary

Instructions:

1. In a large bowl, combine the cooked quinoa, kale, cherry tomatoes, cucumber, red onion, and pumpkin seeds. Toss to mix.
2. To make the dressing, whisk together the tahini, lemon juice, olive oil, maple syrup or honey, garlic, salt, and pepper in a small bowl. Add water, a tablespoon at a time, until you reach the desired consistency.
3. Pour the dressing over the salad and toss to coat evenly.
4. Sprinkle with feta cheese if using.
5. Serve immediately or refrigerate for later.

Benefits: This salad is rich in fiber, antioxidants, and healthy fats. Quinoa provides complete protein, while kale is packed with vitamins A, C, and K. The lemon-tahini dressing adds a zesty and nutritious flavor boost.

---

b. Mediterranean Chickpea Salad

Ingredients:

- 1 can (15 oz) chickpeas, drained and rinsed
- 1 cup cherry tomatoes, halved
- 1/2 cup cucumber, diced

- 1/4 cup red onion, finely chopped
- 1/4 cup Kalamata olives, pitted and sliced
- 1/4 cup crumbled feta cheese
- 1/4 cup fresh parsley, chopped

Dressing:

- 3 tablespoons olive oil
- 2 tablespoons red wine vinegar
- 1 teaspoon dried oregano
- 1 clove garlic, minced
- Salt and pepper to taste

Instructions:

1. In a large bowl, combine the chickpeas, cherry tomatoes, cucumber, red onion, olives, feta cheese, and parsley. Toss to mix.
2. In a small bowl, whisk together the olive oil, red wine vinegar, oregano, garlic, salt, and pepper.
3. Pour the dressing over the salad and toss to coat evenly.
4. Serve immediately or refrigerate for later.

Benefits: Chickpeas are a great source of plant-based protein and fiber. This salad is light yet filling, with plenty of Mediterranean flavors and anti-inflammatory ingredients like olive oil and fresh vegetables.

2. Wholesome Sandwiches and Wraps

a. Grilled Veggie and Hummus Wrap

Ingredients:

- 1 whole-grain or spinach tortilla
- 1/2 cup hummus (store-bought or homemade)
- 1/4 cup roasted red bell peppers, sliced
- 1/4 cup zucchini, grilled and sliced
- 1/4 cup eggplant, grilled and sliced
- 1/4 cup spinach leaves
- 1/4 cup shredded carrots

Instructions:

1. Spread the hummus evenly over the tortilla.
2. Layer the roasted red bell peppers, grilled zucchini, grilled eggplant, spinach leaves, and shredded carrots on top of the hummus.
3. Roll up the tortilla tightly, folding in the sides as you go.
4. Cut the wrap in half and serve immediately.

Benefits: This wrap is packed with colorful vegetables, providing a variety of vitamins, minerals, and antioxidants. Hummus adds protein and healthy fats, making this a balanced and satisfying lunch option.

b. Turkey and Avocado Sandwich

Ingredients:

- 2 slices whole-grain bread
- 4 ounces roasted turkey breast, thinly sliced
- 1/2 avocado, mashed
- 1/4 cup baby spinach leaves
- 2 slices tomato
- 1 tablespoon Dijon mustard
- Salt and pepper to taste

Instructions:

1. Spread the Dijon mustard on one slice of bread.
2. Spread the mashed avocado on the other slice of bread.
3. Layer the turkey, spinach leaves, and tomato slices on top of the avocado.
4. Season with salt and pepper to taste.
5. Top with the slice of bread with mustard.
6. Cut the sandwich in half and serve immediately.

Benefits: This sandwich combines lean protein from the turkey, healthy fats from the avocado, and fiber from the whole-grain bread and spinach. It's a nutritious and delicious option for a quick lunch.

3. Healing Soups and Stews

a. Lentil and Vegetable Soup

Ingredients:

- 1 tablespoon olive oil
- 1 onion, chopped
- 2 carrots, diced
- 2 celery stalks, diced
- 3 cloves garlic, minced
- 1 cup dried lentils, rinsed
- 6 cups vegetable broth
- 1 can (15 oz) diced tomatoes
- 1 teaspoon ground cumin
- 1/2 teaspoon turmeric
- 1/2 teaspoon smoked paprika
- Salt and pepper to taste
- 2 cups spinach leaves
- Juice of 1 lemon
- Fresh parsley, chopped, for garnish

Instructions:

1. In a large pot, heat the olive oil over medium heat. Add the onion, carrots, and celery and sauté until softened, about 5-7 minutes.
2. Add the garlic and cook for another minute.
3. Stir in the lentils, vegetable broth, diced tomatoes, cumin, turmeric, smoked paprika, salt, and pepper.
4. Bring to a boil, then reduce the heat and simmer for 25-30 minutes, or until the lentils are tender.

5. Stir in the spinach leaves and cook until wilted, about 2 minutes.
6. Add the lemon juice and adjust seasoning as needed.
7. Serve hot, garnished with fresh parsley.

Benefits: Lentils are an excellent source of plant-based protein and fiber. This soup is hearty and packed with vegetables and spices known for their anti-inflammatory properties.

---

b. Chicken and Sweet Potato Stew

Ingredients:

- 1 tablespoon olive oil
- 1 onion, chopped
- 2 cloves garlic, minced
- 1 pound boneless, skinless chicken thighs, cut into chunks
- 2 sweet potatoes, peeled and diced
- 1 red bell pepper, chopped
- 1 can (15 oz) diced tomatoes
- 4 cups chicken broth
- 1 teaspoon ground cumin
- 1/2 teaspoon ground coriander
- 1/2 teaspoon ground turmeric
- Salt and pepper to taste
- 1/4 cup fresh cilantro, chopped

Instructions:

1. In a large pot, heat the olive oil over medium heat. Add the onion and cook until softened, about 5 minutes.

2. Add the garlic and cook for another minute.
3. Add the chicken and cook until browned on all sides, about 5-7 minutes.
4. Stir in the sweet potatoes, red bell pepper, diced tomatoes, chicken broth, cumin, coriander, turmeric, salt, and pepper.
5. Bring to a boil, then reduce the heat and simmer for 25-30 minutes, or until the chicken is cooked through and the sweet potatoes are tender.
6. Stir in the fresh cilantro.
7. Serve hot.

Benefits: This stew is rich in protein from the chicken and complex carbohydrates from the sweet potatoes. The spices provide anti-inflammatory benefits, making this a healing and nourishing meal.

4. Easy and Satisfying Midday Meals

a. Baked Salmon with Quinoa and Asparagus

Ingredients:

- 2 salmon fillets
- 1 tablespoon olive oil
- Salt and pepper to taste
- 1 lemon, sliced
- 1 cup quinoa, cooked according to package instructions
- 1 bunch asparagus, trimmed
- 1 tablespoon balsamic vinegar

Instructions:

1. Preheat the oven to 400°F (200°C).
2. Place the salmon fillets on a baking sheet lined with parchment paper. Drizzle with olive oil and season with salt and pepper. Top each fillet with lemon slices.
3. Arrange the asparagus on the same baking sheet, drizzle with olive oil, and season with salt and pepper.
4. Bake for 15-20 minutes, or until the salmon is cooked through and the asparagus is tender.
5. While the salmon and asparagus are baking, cook the quinoa according to package instructions.
6. Serve the baked salmon and asparagus with quinoa, drizzled with balsamic vinegar.

Benefits: Salmon is rich in omega-3 fatty acids, which have strong anti-inflammatory effects. Quinoa provides protein and fiber, and asparagus is a great source of vitamins and minerals.

b. Chickpea and Spinach Stir-Fry

Ingredients:

- 1 can (15 oz) chickpeas, drained and rinsed
- 4 cups fresh spinach leaves
- 1 red bell pepper, sliced
- 1 teaspoon ground cumin
- 1/2 teaspoon smoked paprika
- Salt and pepper to taste
- Juice of 1 lemon
- Fresh cilantro, chopped, for garnish

Instructions:

1. In a large skillet, heat the olive oil over medium heat. Add the onion and cook until softened, about 5 minutes.
2. Add the garlic and cook for another minute until fragrant.
3. Stir in the chickpeas and red bell pepper. Cook until the bell pepper is tender, about 5-7 minutes.
4. Add the spinach, cumin, smoked paprika, salt, and pepper. Stir well to combine.
5. Cook until the spinach is wilted, about 3 minutes.
6. Remove from heat and stir in the lemon juice.
7. Serve hot, garnished with fresh cilantro.

Benefits: This stir-fry is a quick and nutritious option, with chickpeas providing protein and fiber, spinach offering a wealth of vitamins and minerals, and spices adding anti-inflammatory benefits.

With these detailed recipes, you now have a comprehensive selection of lunch options that are both delicious and designed to support the management of GCA and PMR. Each dish emphasizes whole, nutrient-dense ingredients known for their anti-inflammatory properties, ensuring you can enjoy your meals while promoting better health.

CHAPTER 6

DINNER RECIPES

Dinner is often the main meal of the day, providing an opportunity to nourish your body with wholesome, anti-inflammatory foods that aid in the management of Giant Cell Arteritis (GCA) and Polymyalgia Rheumatica (PMR). This chapter offers a variety of dinner recipes that are both delicious and healing.

1. Anti-Inflammatory Main Courses

a. Baked Turmeric Chicken

Ingredients:

- 4 boneless, skinless chicken breasts
- 2 tablespoons olive oil
- 2 teaspoons ground turmeric
- 1 teaspoon ground cumin
- 1 teaspoon ground coriander
- 1 teaspoon paprika
- 1/2 teaspoon ground black pepper
- 1/2 teaspoon sea salt
- Juice of 1 lemon
- 2 cloves garlic, minced

Instructions:

1. Preheat the oven to 375°F (190°C).
2. In a small bowl, mix the olive oil, turmeric, cumin, coriander, paprika, black pepper, sea salt, lemon juice, and garlic to make a marinade.
3. Place the chicken breasts in a baking dish and pour the marinade over them, making sure they are well coated.
4. Cover the dish with aluminum foil and bake for 25-30 minutes, or until the chicken is cooked through and no longer pink in the center.
5. Remove the foil and bake for an additional 5-10 minutes to allow the chicken to brown slightly.
6. Serve hot, garnished with fresh herbs if desired.

Benefits: Turmeric contains curcumin, a powerful anti-inflammatory compound. This dish is also high in protein and seasoned with spices that support overall health.

---

b. Grilled Salmon with Avocado Salsa

Ingredients:

- 4 salmon fillets
- 2 tablespoons olive oil
- Juice of 1 lime
- Salt and pepper to taste

Avocado Salsa:

- 2 ripe avocados, diced

- 1 small red onion, finely chopped
- 1 jalapeño, seeded and finely chopped
- 1/4 cup fresh cilantro, chopped
- Juice of 1 lime
- Salt and pepper to taste

Instructions:

1. Preheat the grill to medium-high heat.
2. Rub the salmon fillets with olive oil, lime juice, salt, and pepper.
3. Grill the salmon for about 4-5 minutes per side, or until it flakes easily with a fork.
4. While the salmon is grilling, prepare the avocado salsa by combining the diced avocados, red onion, jalapeño, cilantro, lime juice, salt, and pepper in a bowl. Mix gently to combine.
5. Serve the grilled salmon topped with the avocado salsa.

Benefits: Salmon is rich in omega-3 fatty acids, which have strong anti-inflammatory properties. The avocado salsa adds healthy fats, fiber, and a refreshing flavor.

---

2. Delicious and Healthy Sides

a. Roasted Brussels Sprouts with Balsamic Glaze

Ingredients:

- 1 pound Brussels sprouts, trimmed and halved
- 2 tablespoons olive oil
- Salt and pepper to taste

- 2 tablespoons balsamic vinegar
- 1 tablespoon honey

Instructions:

1. Preheat the oven to 400°F (200°C).
2. Toss the Brussels sprouts with olive oil, salt, and pepper. Spread them in a single layer on a baking sheet.
3. Roast for 20-25 minutes, or until the Brussels sprouts are golden brown and crispy.
4. While the Brussels sprouts are roasting, combine the balsamic vinegar and honey in a small saucepan. Bring to a simmer and cook until reduced and slightly thickened, about 5 minutes.
5. Drizzle the balsamic glaze over the roasted Brussels sprouts before serving.

Benefits: Brussels sprouts are high in fiber, vitamins, and antioxidants. The balsamic glaze adds a touch of sweetness and depth of flavor.

---

b. Quinoa and Roasted Vegetable Salad

Ingredients:

- 1 cup quinoa, rinsed and drained
- 2 cups water or vegetable broth
- 1 red bell pepper, diced
- 1 zucchini, diced
- 1 red onion, diced
- 2 tablespoons olive oil

- Salt and pepper to taste
- 1/4 cup fresh parsley, chopped
- Juice of 1 lemon

Instructions:

1. Preheat the oven to 400°F (200°C).
2. Toss the diced red bell pepper, zucchini, and red onion with olive oil, salt, and pepper. Spread them on a baking sheet and roast for 20-25 minutes, or until tender and lightly browned.
3. While the vegetables are roasting, bring the water or vegetable broth to a boil in a medium saucepan. Add the quinoa, reduce the heat, and simmer for 15 minutes, or until the quinoa is cooked and the liquid is absorbed.
4. Fluff the quinoa with a fork and transfer it to a large bowl.
5. Add the roasted vegetables, fresh parsley, and lemon juice to the quinoa. Toss to combine.
6. Serve warm or at room temperature.

Benefits: Quinoa is a complete protein and provides essential amino acids. The roasted vegetables add vitamins, minerals, and a variety of flavors.

---

3. One-Pot and Slow Cooker Meals

a. Slow Cooker Chicken and Sweet Potato Curry

Ingredients:

- 1 pound boneless, skinless chicken thighs, cut into chunks
- 2 sweet potatoes, peeled and diced

- 1 onion, chopped
- 3 cloves garlic, minced
- 1 can (15 oz) coconut milk
- 1 can (15 oz) diced tomatoes
- 2 tablespoons curry powder
- 1 teaspoon ground turmeric
- 1 teaspoon ground cumin
- Salt and pepper to taste
- Fresh cilantro, chopped, for garnish

Instructions:

1. Place the chicken, sweet potatoes, onion, and garlic in the slow cooker.
2. Add the coconut milk, diced tomatoes, curry powder, turmeric, cumin, salt, and pepper. Stir to combine.
3. Cover and cook on low for 6-8 hours, or on high for 3-4 hours, until the chicken and sweet potatoes are tender.
4. Serve hot, garnished with fresh cilantro.

Benefits: This curry is rich in anti-inflammatory spices and healthy fats from the coconut milk. It's a comforting and nutritious meal that's easy to prepare.

---

b. One-Pot Lemon Garlic Shrimp and Rice

Ingredients:

- 1 tablespoon olive oil
- 1 onion, chopped
- 3 cloves garlic, minced

- 1 cup long-grain rice
- 2 cups vegetable or chicken broth
- 1 pound shrimp, peeled and deveined
- Juice of 1 lemon
- Zest of 1 lemon
- 1/4 cup fresh parsley, chopped
- Salt and pepper to taste

Instructions:

1. In a large pot, heat the olive oil over medium heat. Add the onion and cook until softened, about 5 minutes.
2. Add the garlic and cook for another minute.
3. Stir in the rice and cook for 1-2 minutes, until lightly toasted.
4. Pour in the broth and bring to a boil. Reduce the heat, cover, and simmer for 15-18 minutes, or until the rice is tender and the liquid is absorbed.
5. Stir in the shrimp, lemon juice, and lemon zest. Cook for another 5 minutes, or until the shrimp are pink and cooked through.
6. Remove from heat and stir in the fresh parsley. Season with salt and pepper to taste.
7. Serve hot.

Benefits: This one-pot meal is easy to prepare and clean up. Shrimp is a low-calorie source of protein, and the lemon and garlic add a burst of flavor and additional health benefits.

4. Comfort Food with a Healing Twist

a. Cauliflower Mac and Cheese

Ingredients:

- 1 head cauliflower, cut into florets
- 1 cup unsweetened almond milk
- 1/2 cup nutritional yeast
- 1/4 cup cashews, soaked in hot water for 30 minutes and drained
- 2 tablespoons olive oil
- 1 tablespoon Dijon mustard
- 1 teaspoon garlic powder
- 1 teaspoon onion powder
- Salt and pepper to taste
- Fresh chives, chopped, for garnish

Instructions:

1. Preheat the oven to 375°F (190°C).
2. Bring a large pot of water to a boil. Add the cauliflower florets and cook until tender, about 5-7 minutes. Drain and set aside.
3. In a blender, combine the almond milk, nutritional yeast, soaked cashews, olive oil, Dijon mustard, garlic powder, onion powder, salt, and pepper. Blend until smooth and creamy.
4. Place the cooked cauliflower in a baking dish and pour the sauce over the top. Toss to coat the cauliflower evenly.
5. Bake for 15-20 minutes, or until the sauce is bubbly and slightly golden on top.
6. Serve hot, garnished with fresh chives.

Benefits: This cauliflower mac and cheese is a healthier, dairy-free version of the classic comfort food. Cauliflower is rich in vitamins and fiber, and the cashew-based sauce provides healthy fats and protein.

b. Turkey and Vegetable Shepherd's Pie

Ingredients:

- 2 tablespoons tomato paste
- 1 teaspoon Worcestershire sauce
- 1 teaspoon dried thyme
- Salt and pepper to taste
- 4 cups mashed potatoes (prepared)
- Fresh parsley, chopped, for garnish

Instructions:

1. Preheat the oven to 375°F (190°C).
2. In a large skillet, heat olive oil over medium heat. Add the chopped onion and cook until softened, about 5 minutes.
3. Add the minced garlic and cook for another minute until fragrant.
4. Add the ground turkey to the skillet and cook until browned, breaking it up with a spoon as it cooks.
5. Stir in the diced carrots, peas, and corn. Cook for an additional 5 minutes.
6. In a small bowl, whisk together the vegetable broth, tomato paste, Worcestershire sauce, dried thyme, salt, and pepper.
7. Pour the broth mixture over the turkey and vegetables in the skillet. Stir well to combine. Simmer for 5-10 minutes until the mixture thickens slightly.
8. Transfer the turkey and vegetable mixture to a baking dish.

9. Spread the mashed potatoes evenly over the top of the turkey mixture.
10. Bake for 25-30 minutes, or until the mashed potatoes are lightly golden on top.
11. Garnish with fresh parsley before serving.

Benefits: This turkey and vegetable shepherd's pie is a comforting and nutritious dish that's perfect for a cozy dinner. It's packed with lean protein, vegetables, and hearty flavors.

With these diverse dinner recipes, you have a range of options to enjoy nutritious and satisfying meals while managing GCA and PMR. Each dish is designed to be flavorful, comforting, and supportive of your overall health and well-being.

CHAPTER 7

SNACKS AND APPETIZERS

Snacks and appetizers are important parts of your daily nutrition, especially when managing Giant Cell Arteritis (GCA) and Polymyalgia Rheumatica (PMR). They help maintain energy levels and prevent inflammation flare-ups. This chapter provides a variety of quick, healthy, and delicious options that are easy to prepare and enjoy.

1. Quick and Healthy Snacks

a. Greek Yogurt and Berry Parfait

Ingredients:

- 1 cup Greek yogurt (plain, unsweetened)
- 1/2 cup mixed berries (blueberries, strawberries, raspberries)
- 2 tablespoons honey or maple syrup
- 1/4 cup granola (optional)
- Fresh mint leaves for garnish

Instructions:

1. In a glass or bowl, layer half of the Greek yogurt.
2. Add a layer of mixed berries.
3. Drizzle with honey or maple syrup.
4. Add another layer of Greek yogurt and berries.

5. Top with granola if desired.
6. Garnish with fresh mint leaves.
7. Serve immediately.

Benefits: Greek yogurt is high in protein and probiotics, which support gut health. Berries are rich in antioxidants and vitamins, making this a refreshing and nutritious snack.

b. Apple Slices with Almond Butter

Ingredients:

- 1 large apple (any variety), cored and sliced
- 2 tablespoons almond butter
- 1 teaspoon chia seeds (optional)
- 1 teaspoon ground cinnamon (optional)

Instructions:

1. Arrange the apple slices on a plate.
2. Spread almond butter evenly over each slice.
3. Sprinkle with chia seeds and ground cinnamon if desired.
4. Serve immediately.

Benefits: This snack combines fiber-rich apples with protein and healthy fats from almond butter, providing sustained energy and satiety. Chia seeds add omega-3 fatty acids, and cinnamon has anti-inflammatory properties.

2. Anti-Inflammatory Dips and Spreads

a. Classic Hummus

Ingredients:

- 1/4 cup fresh lemon juice (about 1 large lemon)
- 1/4 cup tahini
- 1 small garlic clove, minced
- 2 tablespoons extra-virgin olive oil, plus more for serving
- 1/2 teaspoon ground cumin
- Salt to taste
- 2 to 3 tablespoons water
- Paprika for garnish
- Fresh parsley for garnish

Instructions:

1. In a food processor, combine the tahini and lemon juice. Process for 1 minute until smooth and creamy.
2. Add the minced garlic, olive oil, cumin, and salt to the mixture. Process for another 30 seconds, scraping down the sides of the bowl as needed.
3. Add half of the chickpeas to the food processor and process for 1 minute. Scrape down the sides of the bowl and add the remaining chickpeas. Process until smooth, about 1-2 minutes.
4. If the hummus is too thick, add 2 to 3 tablespoons of water and process until the desired consistency is reached.
5. Transfer the hummus to a serving bowl, drizzle with olive oil, and sprinkle with paprika and fresh parsley.
6. Serve with fresh vegetables, whole-grain crackers, or pita bread.

Benefits: Hummus is an excellent source of plant-based protein and fiber. Chickpeas and tahini are rich in nutrients that support heart health and have anti-inflammatory properties.

---

b. Avocado and Edamame Dip

Ingredients:

- 1 ripe avocado, peeled and pitted
- 1 cup shelled edamame (thawed if frozen)
- 1 small garlic clove
- 2 tablespoons lime juice
- 2 tablespoons olive oil
- Salt and pepper to taste
- 1/4 cup fresh cilantro, chopped

Instructions:

1. In a food processor, combine the avocado, edamame, garlic, lime juice, and olive oil. Process until smooth.
2. Season with salt and pepper to taste.
3. Transfer the dip to a serving bowl and stir in the fresh cilantro.
4. Serve with fresh vegetables, whole-grain crackers, or use as a spread for sandwiches and wraps.

Benefits: Avocados and edamame are rich in healthy fats, fiber, and protein. This dip provides a creamy, nutrient-dense snack that's perfect for fighting inflammation.

3. Nourishing Small Bites

a. Stuffed Mini Bell Peppers

Ingredients:

- 1 pint mini bell peppers, halved and seeded
- 1 cup ricotta cheese
- 1/4 cup fresh basil, chopped
- 2 tablespoons fresh lemon juice
- 1 teaspoon lemon zest
- Salt and pepper to taste
- 1/4 cup pine nuts, toasted

Instructions:

1. In a medium bowl, combine the ricotta cheese, basil, lemon juice, lemon zest, salt, and pepper. Mix well.
2. Spoon the ricotta mixture into the halved mini bell peppers.
3. Arrange the stuffed peppers on a serving platter.
4. Sprinkle with toasted pine nuts.
5. Serve immediately.

Benefits: These small bites are packed with flavor and nutrients. Bell peppers are high in vitamins A and C, while ricotta cheese provides protein and calcium. Pine nuts add healthy fats and a satisfying crunch.

b. Cucumber and Smoked Salmon Bites

Ingredients:

- 1 large cucumber, sliced into rounds
- 4 ounces smoked salmon, sliced into small pieces
- 1/4 cup cream cheese or Greek yogurt
- 1 tablespoon fresh dill, chopped
- 1 tablespoon capers, drained
- Freshly ground black pepper

Instructions:

1. Spread a small amount of cream cheese or Greek yogurt on each cucumber slice.
2. Top each slice with a piece of smoked salmon.
3. Garnish with fresh dill, capers, and a sprinkle of black pepper.
4. Serve immediately.

Benefits: These bites are light yet satisfying, providing a good source of omega-3 fatty acids from the smoked salmon, which help reduce inflammation. Cucumbers add hydration and a refreshing crunch.

4. Energy-Boosting Nibbles

a. Nut and Seed Energy Bars

Ingredients:

- 1 cup rolled oats
- 1/2 cup almonds, chopped
- 1/2 cup sunflower seeds
- 1/4 cup chia seeds
- 1/4 cup flaxseeds
- 1/2 cup dried cranberries
- 1/2 cup honey or maple syrup
- 1/2 cup almond butter
- 1 teaspoon vanilla extract

Instructions:

1. Preheat the oven to 350°F (175°C). Line a baking dish with parchment paper.
2. In a large bowl, combine the oats, almonds, sunflower seeds, chia seeds, flaxseeds, and dried cranberries.
3. In a small saucepan, heat the honey or maple syrup and almond butter over medium heat until smooth. Remove from heat and stir in the vanilla extract.
4. Pour the wet mixture over the dry ingredients and stir until well combined.
5. Press the mixture firmly into the prepared baking dish.
6. Bake for 15-20 minutes, or until the edges are golden brown.
7. Let cool completely before cutting into bars.
8. Store in an airtight container.

Benefits: These energy bars are packed with nuts and seeds, providing healthy fats, protein, and fiber. They make a perfect on-the-go snack that keeps you energized and full.

---

b. Dark Chocolate and Nut Clusters

Ingredients:

- 1 cup dark chocolate chips (70% cacao or higher)
- 1/2 cup almonds, chopped
- 1/2 cup walnuts, chopped
- 1/4 cup dried cherries or cranberries

Instructions:

1. Line a baking sheet with parchment paper.
2. Melt the dark chocolate chips in a double boiler or in the microwave, stirring until smooth.
3. Stir in the chopped almonds, walnuts, and dried cherries or cranberries.
4. Drop spoonfuls of the mixture onto the prepared baking sheet.
5. Let the clusters cool and harden completely at room temperature, or refrigerate until set.
6. Store in an airtight container.

Benefits: Dark chocolate is rich in antioxidants, and the nuts provide healthy fats and protein. This snack satisfies sweet cravings while offering nutritional benefits.

These snacks and appetizers provide a range of nutritious and delicious options that support anti-inflammatory diets, helping to manage GCA and PMR. Each recipe is designed to be quick, easy, and packed with health benefits.

CHAPTER 8

DESSERTS AND TREATS

Desserts and treats can be part of a healthy diet, especially when they are made with anti-inflammatory ingredients. This chapter offers a variety of guilt-free, fruit-based, and simple desserts that satisfy your sweet tooth while supporting your health.

1. Guilt-Free Sweet Treats

a. Dark Chocolate Avocado Mousse

Ingredients:

- 2 ripe avocados, peeled and pitted
- 1/4 cup cocoa powder
- 1/4 cup maple syrup or honey
- 1/4 cup almond milk (or any non-dairy milk)
- 1 teaspoon vanilla extract
- A pinch of sea salt
- Fresh berries and mint leaves for garnish

Instructions:

1. In a food processor, combine the avocados, cocoa powder, maple syrup, almond milk, vanilla extract, and sea salt. Process until smooth and creamy.
2. Taste and adjust sweetness if necessary.

3. Divide the mousse into serving bowls and refrigerate for at least 30 minutes before serving.
4. Garnish with fresh berries and mint leaves.

Benefits: This mousse is rich and creamy, with avocados providing healthy fats and antioxidants. The dark chocolate adds a deep flavor and is also high in antioxidants.

---

b. Coconut Chia Pudding

Ingredients:

- 1 cup coconut milk (from a carton, not a can)
- 1/4 cup chia seeds
- 2 tablespoons maple syrup or honey
- 1 teaspoon vanilla extract
- Fresh fruit for topping

Instructions:

1. In a bowl, whisk together the coconut milk, chia seeds, maple syrup, and vanilla extract.
2. Cover and refrigerate for at least 4 hours or overnight, until the mixture thickens to a pudding-like consistency.
3. Stir well before serving, and top with fresh fruit.

Benefits: Chia seeds are packed with omega-3 fatty acids, fiber, and protein. This pudding is a light and refreshing dessert that supports digestive health.

2. Fruit-Based Desserts

a. Baked Apples with Cinnamon and Walnuts

Ingredients:

- 4 large apples, cored
- 1/4 cup chopped walnuts
- 2 tablespoons raisins
- 2 tablespoons maple syrup or honey
- 1 teaspoon ground cinnamon
- 1/2 teaspoon ground nutmeg

Instructions:

1. Preheat the oven to 350°F (175°C).
2. Place the cored apples in a baking dish.
3. In a small bowl, combine the chopped walnuts, raisins, maple syrup, ground cinnamon, and nutmeg.
4. Stuff the mixture into the center of each apple.
5. Add a small amount of water to the bottom of the baking dish to prevent sticking.
6. Bake for 30-35 minutes, or until the apples are tender.
7. Serve warm, optionally with a dollop of Greek yogurt.

Benefits: Apples are high in fiber and vitamins, and the spices used have anti-inflammatory properties. This dessert is both comforting and nutritious.

b. Grilled Peaches with Honey and Yogurt

Ingredients:

- 4 ripe peaches, halved and pitted
- 2 tablespoons honey
- 1 cup Greek yogurt
- Fresh mint leaves for garnish

Instructions:

1. Preheat the grill to medium-high heat.
2. Place the peach halves on the grill, cut side down, and cook for 3-4 minutes, or until grill marks appear and the peaches are slightly softened.
3. Remove from the grill and drizzle with honey.
4. Serve each peach half with a spoonful of Greek yogurt.
5. Garnish with fresh mint leaves.

Benefits: Peaches are rich in vitamins A and C, while Greek yogurt adds protein and probiotics. This simple dessert is refreshing and healthy.

3. Anti-Inflammatory Baked Goods

a. Almond Flour Blueberry Muffins

Ingredients:

- 2 cups almond flour
- 1/2 teaspoon baking soda
- 1/4 teaspoon salt
- 2 eggs
- 1/4 cup honey or maple syrup
- 1/4 cup almond milk
- 1 teaspoon vanilla extract
- 1 cup fresh or frozen blueberries

Instructions:

1. Preheat the oven to 350°F (175°C) and line a muffin tin with paper liners.
2. In a large bowl, whisk together the almond flour, baking soda, and salt.
3. In a separate bowl, beat the eggs and mix in the honey, almond milk, and vanilla extract.
4. Add the wet ingredients to the dry ingredients and mix until just combined.
5. Gently fold in the blueberries.
6. Divide the batter evenly among the muffin cups.
7. Bake for 20-25 minutes, or until a toothpick inserted into the center comes out clean.
8. Allow the muffins to cool before serving.

Benefits: Almond flour is a great alternative to wheat flour, providing protein, healthy fats, and a lower glycemic index. Blueberries add antioxidants and natural sweetness.

---

b. Turmeric Ginger Cookies

Ingredients:

- 1 1/2 cups oat flour
- 1/2 teaspoon baking soda
- 1/2 teaspoon ground turmeric
- 1/2 teaspoon ground ginger
- 1/4 teaspoon salt
- 1/2 cup coconut oil, melted
- 1/2 cup coconut sugar
- 1 egg
- 1 teaspoon vanilla extract

Instructions:

1. Preheat the oven to 350°F (175°C) and line a baking sheet with parchment paper.
2. In a medium bowl, whisk together the oat flour, baking soda, turmeric, ginger, and salt.
3. In a separate bowl, mix the melted coconut oil and coconut sugar until well combined.
4. Beat in the egg and vanilla extract.
5. Gradually add the dry ingredients to the wet ingredients, mixing until a dough forms.
6. Drop spoonfuls of the dough onto the prepared baking sheet.
7. Bake for 10-12 minutes, or until the edges are golden brown.

8. Allow the cookies to cool on the baking sheet for a few minutes before transferring to a wire rack to cool completely.

Benefits: These cookies incorporate anti-inflammatory spices like turmeric and ginger, making them a healthy treat option. Oat flour is high in fiber and provides a gluten-free alternative to wheat flour.

4. Simple and Satisfying Desserts

a. Banana Nice Cream

Ingredients:

- 4 ripe bananas, sliced and frozen
- 1 teaspoon vanilla extract
- 1 tablespoon almond milk (optional)
- Dark chocolate shavings (optional)

Instructions:

1. Place the frozen banana slices in a food processor.
2. Blend until the bananas break down and become creamy. You may need to stop and scrape down the sides a few times.
3. Add the vanilla extract and blend until smooth. If the mixture is too thick, add almond milk one tablespoon at a time.
4. Serve immediately, topped with dark chocolate shavings if desired.

Benefits: This "nice cream" is a dairy-free, low-calorie alternative to traditional ice cream. Bananas are rich in potassium and provide natural sweetness.

---

b. Berry Chia Seed Jam

Ingredients:

- 2 cups mixed berries (fresh or frozen)
- 2 tablespoons chia seeds
- 1-2 tablespoons honey or maple syrup
- 1 teaspoon lemon juice

Instructions:

1. In a small saucepan, cook the berries over medium heat until they break down and become syrupy, about 5-10 minutes.
2. Use a fork or potato masher to mash the berries to your desired consistency.
3. Stir in the chia seeds, honey or maple syrup, and lemon juice.
4. Remove from heat and let the mixture sit for 5-10 minutes to thicken.
5. Transfer to a jar and refrigerate. The jam will continue to thicken as it cools.
6. Serve on toast, yogurt, or as a topping for desserts.

Benefits: This chia seed jam is a healthy alternative to store-bought jams, which often contain added sugars and preservatives. Berries and chia seeds provide antioxidants, fiber, and omega-3 fatty acids.

These dessert recipes offer a variety of healthy, anti-inflammatory options to satisfy your sweet cravings while supporting your overall health and well-being. Each treat is designed to be delicious, nutritious, and easy to make.

CHAPTER 9

MEAL PLANS AND DIETARY STRATEGIES

Managing Giant Cell Arteritis (GCA) and Polymyalgia Rheumatica (PMR) effectively involves careful planning and dietary strategies. This chapter provides comprehensive meal plans, customization tips, strategies for dining out, and guidance on monitoring and adjusting your diet.

1. Weekly Meal Plans for Beginners

Starting a new diet can be overwhelming, but having a structured plan makes it easier. Below are sample meal plans for a week, designed to provide balanced nutrition while managing inflammation.

Week 1 Meal Plan

Day 1:

- **Breakfast:** Greek Yogurt and Berry Parfait
- **Snack:** Apple Slices with Almond Butter
- **Lunch:** Quinoa and Chickpea Salad
- **Snack:** Hummus with Carrot Sticks
- **Dinner:** Baked Salmon with Roasted Vegetables
- **Dessert:** Dark Chocolate Avocado Mousse

Day 2:

- **Breakfast:** Almond Flour Blueberry Muffins
- **Snack:** Cucumber and Smoked Salmon Bites
- **Lunch:** Lentil Soup
- **Snack:** Nut and Seed Energy Bars
- **Dinner:** Turkey and Vegetable Shepherd's Pie
- **Dessert:** Baked Apples with Cinnamon and Walnuts

Day 3:

- **Breakfast:** Turmeric Ginger Smoothie
- **Snack:** Coconut Chia Pudding
- **Lunch:** Grilled Chicken Wrap with Avocado
- **Snack:** Stuffed Mini Bell Peppers
- **Dinner:** Grilled Peaches with Honey and Yogurt
- **Dessert:** Berry Chia Seed Jam on Whole-Grain Toast

Day 4:

- **Breakfast:** Oatmeal with Fresh Fruit and Nuts
- **Snack:** Dark Chocolate and Nut Clusters
- **Lunch:** Spinach and Feta Stuffed Peppers
- **Snack:** Avocado and Edamame Dip with Veggie Sticks
- **Dinner:** Zucchini Noodles with Pesto and Shrimp
- **Dessert:** Banana Nice Cream

Day 5:

- **Breakfast:** Whole Grain Pancakes with Berries
- **Snack:** Greek Yogurt with Honey and Walnuts
- **Lunch:** Hearty Vegetable Stew
- **Snack:** Almond Butter on Rice Cakes

- **Dinner:** Chicken and Quinoa Stir-Fry
- **Dessert:** Coconut Chia Pudding

Day 6:

- **Breakfast:** Smoothie Bowl with Mixed Fruits and Seeds
- **Snack:** Baked Sweet Potato Chips
- **Lunch:** Kale and Quinoa Salad
- **Snack:** Dark Chocolate Avocado Mousse
- **Dinner:** Turkey Chili
- **Dessert:** Almond Flour Blueberry Muffins

Day 7:

- **Breakfast:** Chia Seed Pudding with Mango
- **Snack:** Fresh Vegetable Sticks with Hummus
- **Lunch:** Baked Cod with Lemon and Asparagus
- **Snack:** Nut and Seed Energy Bars
- **Dinner:** Grilled Vegetables and Tofu
- **Dessert:** Baked Apples with Cinnamon and Walnuts

---

2. Customizing Your Diet Plan

Everyone's dietary needs and preferences are different. Customizing your diet plan involves understanding your body's reactions, preferences, and nutritional requirements.

Assess Your Needs:

- **Identify Trigger Foods:** Keep a food diary to note any foods that cause symptoms or discomfort.

- **Understand Your Nutritional Needs:** Consider any deficiencies or additional requirements, such as protein for muscle maintenance or omega-3 fatty acids for inflammation.

Personal Preferences:

- **Flavor and Texture Preferences:** Adjust recipes to match your taste. For example, swap ingredients in smoothies or salads to suit your palate.
- **Cultural and Dietary Restrictions:** Customize meal plans to accommodate dietary restrictions (e.g., gluten-free, vegetarian, vegan).

Portion Control:

- Adjust portions based on your energy requirements, activity levels, and weight management goals.

Flexibility:

- Allow flexibility in meal plans to accommodate unexpected events or cravings. Choose healthier alternatives when necessary.

3. Tips for Dining Out and Social Eating

Maintaining your diet while dining out or at social events can be challenging. Here are some strategies to help you stay on track.

Before Dining Out:

- **Research Menus:** Check the restaurant's menu online and decide on healthier options in advance.
- **Eat a Small Snack:** Have a small, healthy snack before you go out to avoid overeating.

At the Restaurant:

- **Choose Wisely:** Opt for grilled, baked, or steamed dishes instead of fried. Ask for dressings and sauces on the side.
- **Control Portions:** Consider sharing dishes or taking half your meal home.
- **Customize Orders:** Don't hesitate to ask for modifications, such as extra vegetables or a side salad instead of fries.

At Social Events:

- **Bring a Dish:** Offer to bring a healthy dish that you can enjoy and share with others.
- **Survey the Options:** Look at all the available foods before choosing what to eat. Fill your plate with healthy options first.
- **Stay Hydrated:** Drink water throughout the event to stay hydrated and reduce the temptation to overeat.

4. Monitoring and Adjusting Your Diet

Continually monitoring your diet and making necessary adjustments is crucial for long-term success in managing GCA and PMR.

Keep a Food Journal:

- **Track Meals and Symptoms:** Note what you eat and any symptoms you experience. This helps identify trigger foods.
- **Monitor Nutrient Intake:** Ensure you're getting a balanced diet with adequate vitamins, minerals, protein, and healthy fats.

Regular Check-Ins:

- **Assess Progress:** Regularly evaluate how your diet affects your symptoms and overall well-being.
- **Adjust Portions and Ingredients:** Modify portion sizes or ingredients based on your energy levels, weight changes, and symptom management.

Consult Healthcare Providers:

- **Regular Consultations:** Have regular check-ins with your healthcare provider or a registered dietitian to discuss your progress and any necessary dietary adjustments.
- **Laboratory Tests:** Periodically check your blood work to monitor inflammation markers and nutrient levels.

Stay Informed:

- **Educate Yourself:** Stay updated on the latest research and dietary recommendations for managing GCA and PMR.

- **Join Support Groups:** Connect with others who have similar conditions for support, tips, and new recipes.

By following these meal plans and dietary strategies, you can effectively manage GCA and PMR while enjoying delicious and nutritious foods. Consistency and adaptability are key to maintaining a healthy and balanced diet.

CHAPTER 10

LIFESTYLE TIPS FOR MANAGING GCA AND PMR

Managing Giant Cell Arteritis (GCA) and Polymyalgia Rheumatica (PMR) involves more than just dietary changes; lifestyle modifications are crucial for effectively managing symptoms and improving overall well-being. This chapter offers detailed and practical insights into incorporating exercise, managing stress, prioritizing sleep, and building a support system.

1. The Role of Exercise and Physical Activity

Exercise plays a vital role in managing symptoms, improving mobility, and enhancing overall health for individuals with GCA and PMR. Here's how to incorporate exercise into your routine:

Types of Exercise:

- **Aerobic Exercise:** Engage in low-impact activities such as walking, swimming, or cycling to improve cardiovascular health and stamina.
- **Strength Training:** Incorporate resistance exercises using light weights or resistance bands to maintain muscle strength and joint flexibility.
- **Flexibility Exercises:** Perform gentle stretching exercises to improve range of motion and reduce stiffness.

Exercise Guidelines:

- **Start Slowly:** Begin with short, low-intensity sessions and gradually increase duration and intensity as tolerated.
- **Listen to Your Body:** Pay attention to how your body responds to exercise and adjust intensity or duration accordingly.
- **Be Consistent:** Aim for regular exercise sessions several times per week to reap the benefits.

2. Stress Management and Mindfulness Practices

Chronic stress can exacerbate symptoms of GCA and PMR. Incorporating stress management techniques and mindfulness practices can help reduce stress levels and improve overall well-being:

Stress Reduction Techniques:

- **Deep Breathing:** Practice deep breathing exercises to promote relaxation and reduce tension.
- **Mindfulness Meditation:** Set aside time each day for mindfulness meditation to cultivate awareness and calmness.
- **Progressive Muscle Relaxation:** Learn to systematically tense and relax muscle groups to release physical tension.
- **Yoga or Tai Chi:** Engage in gentle, mind-body exercises like yoga or tai chi to reduce stress and improve flexibility.

Stress Management Tips:

- **Prioritize Self-Care:** Make time for activities that bring you joy and relaxation, such as reading, gardening, or spending time with loved ones.
- **Set Boundaries:** Learn to say no to additional commitments or obligations that cause undue stress.
- **Seek Support:** Reach out to friends, family members, or a therapist for support and guidance during stressful times.

3. Importance of Sleep and Rest

Quality sleep is essential for managing symptoms and promoting overall health. Follow these tips to improve sleep quality:

Sleep Hygiene Tips:

- **Establish a Routine:** Maintain a consistent sleep schedule by going to bed and waking up at the same time each day.
- **Create a Relaxing Environment:** Make your bedroom conducive to sleep by keeping it dark, quiet, and cool.
- **Limit Stimulants:** Avoid caffeine, nicotine, and electronic devices before bedtime, as they can interfere with sleep.
- **Practice Relaxation Techniques:** Wind down before bed with relaxation techniques such as reading, taking a warm bath, or practicing deep breathing exercises.

Rest and Recovery:

- **Listen to Your Body:** Pay attention to signals of fatigue or pain, and allow yourself to rest when needed.

- **Pace Yourself:** Break tasks into manageable chunks and take regular breaks to prevent overexertion.
- **Prioritize Restful Activities:** Incorporate relaxation into your daily routine, whether it's through meditation, gentle stretching, or simply taking a quiet moment to yourself.

---

4. Building a Support System

Having a strong support system can provide emotional, practical, and social support when managing GCA and PMR:

Types of Support:

- **Family and Friends:** Lean on loved ones for emotional support, companionship, and assistance with daily tasks.
- **Healthcare Providers:** Build a collaborative relationship with your healthcare team, including your primary care physician, rheumatologist, and other specialists involved in your care.
- **Support Groups:** Join local or online support groups for individuals living with GCA and PMR to connect with others, share experiences, and gain valuable insights and resources.
- **Therapy:** Consider individual or group therapy to process emotions, learn coping strategies, and develop resilience in managing chronic health conditions.

Communication and Advocacy:

- **Open Communication:** Communicate openly with your support network about your needs, challenges, and goals.

- **Educate Others:** Help educate family, friends, and caregivers about GCA and PMR to foster understanding and support.
- **Advocate for Yourself:** Take an active role in your healthcare decisions, ask questions, and advocate for the support and resources you need to manage your condition effectively.

By incorporating these detailed lifestyle tips into your daily routine, you can effectively manage GCA and PMR while enhancing your overall quality of life. Consistency, patience, and self-care are key to achieving long-term well-being.

CHAPTER 11

FREQUENTLY ASKED QUESTIONS

This chapter addresses common dietary concerns, provides guidance on adapting recipes for special diets, and offers troubleshooting tips for success when following the Giant Cell Arteritis (GCA) Diet Cookbook. Let's dive into each subsection separately:

Common Dietary Concerns

Addressing common dietary concerns is essential when managing Giant Cell Arteritis (GCA) and Polymyalgia Rheumatica (PMR) through dietary changes. Let's explore these concerns in greater detail:

1. Flavorful Meals:
The GCA Diet Cookbook prioritizes flavorful meals without compromising health goals. Through careful selection of herbs, spices, and nutrient-rich ingredients, each recipe is designed to delight your taste buds while supporting your well-being. From vibrant salads bursting with fresh produce to hearty soups and flavorful entrees, there's a diverse array of delicious options to explore. The cookbook encourages creativity in the kitchen, allowing you to enjoy a variety of flavors and textures while adhering to your dietary guidelines.

2. Avoiding Trigger Foods:
While following the GCA Diet Cookbook, it's crucial to be mindful

of potential trigger foods that may exacerbate symptoms of inflammation. Processed foods, refined sugars, trans fats, and high-sodium meals are common culprits known to contribute to inflammation and discomfort. By being attentive to your body's responses and keeping a food journal, you can identify specific foods that may trigger adverse reactions and adjust your diet accordingly. Additionally, consulting with a healthcare professional or registered dietitian can provide personalized guidance on navigating potential trigger foods and making informed dietary choices.

3. Nutritional Adequacy:
Ensuring that your diet meets your nutritional needs is fundamental for supporting overall health and managing symptoms of GCA and PMR. The GCA Diet Cookbook emphasizes the importance of a well-balanced diet rich in essential nutrients. To achieve optimal nutrition, focus on incorporating a diverse array of colorful fruits, vegetables, whole grains, lean proteins, and healthy fats into your meals. Paying attention to portion sizes, staying hydrated, and considering the use of supplements under the guidance of a healthcare professional can further support your nutritional goals. Additionally, periodic assessment of your dietary intake and monitoring of key nutrients can help identify any potential deficiencies and inform adjustments to your meal plan.

Q: Can I still enjoy flavorful meals while following the GCA Diet Cookbook? A: Absolutely! The recipes in this cookbook are crafted to be both delicious and health-supportive. By utilizing a diverse array of herbs, spices, and wholesome ingredients, you can create meals bursting with flavor while adhering to your dietary guidelines.

Q: Are there any foods I should avoid completely? A: While the GCA Diet Cookbook emphasizes anti-inflammatory ingredients, it's essential to be mindful of individual tolerances. Some individuals may find certain foods exacerbate symptoms of inflammation. Common trigger foods include processed foods, refined sugars, and excessive alcohol. It's advisable to listen to your body and identify any potential trigger foods through a process of elimination.

Q: How can I ensure I'm getting enough nutrients on this diet? A: Maintaining a well-rounded and varied diet is key to meeting your nutritional needs while following the GCA Diet Cookbook. Aim to incorporate a diverse range of fruits, vegetables, whole grains, lean proteins, and healthy fats into your meals. If you have specific concerns about meeting your nutritional requirements, consider consulting with a registered dietitian for personalized guidance.

---

2. Adapting Recipes for Special Diets

For individuals with special dietary needs, the GCA Diet Cookbook offers flexibility and adaptability. Whether you have food allergies, intolerances, or follow a specific dietary pattern such as vegetarian, vegan, or low-carb, many recipes can be modified to suit your requirements. For example, dairy-free alternatives can be substituted for dairy products, gluten-free flours for wheat flour, and plant-based proteins for animal products. Additionally, recipes can be adjusted to accommodate preferences for lower sodium, sugar, or fat content. Experimenting with alternative ingredients and exploring diverse cooking techniques allows you to tailor recipes to meet your individual dietary needs while still enjoying flavorful and nutritious

Q: I have food allergies. Can I still use the recipes in this cookbook? A: Absolutely! Many recipes in the GCA Diet Cookbook can be easily adapted to accommodate food allergies or intolerances. For example, you can substitute dairy-free alternatives for dairy products, gluten-free flours for wheat flour, or omit ingredients that trigger allergies.

Q: Are there options for vegetarians or vegans in this cookbook? A: Yes! Several recipes in this cookbook are vegetarian or vegan-friendly, and others can be easily modified by substituting plant-based ingredients for animal products. Look for recipes labeled as vegetarian or vegan, and feel free to experiment with plant-based alternatives to suit your dietary preferences.

Q: I follow a low-carb diet. Can I still incorporate these recipes into my meal plan? A: Absolutely! While some recipes in this cookbook may contain carbohydrates, there are plenty of options suitable for individuals following a low-carb diet. Focus on recipes that emphasize protein, healthy fats, and non-starchy vegetables, and adjust portion sizes as needed to align with your dietary preferences.

3. Troubleshooting and Tips for Success

Embarking on a dietary journey can sometimes come with challenges and obstacles. However, with the right strategies and tips, you can overcome these hurdles and achieve success. Common challenges may include difficulty finding specific ingredients, sticking to the meal plan, or not seeing the expected results. To troubleshoot these issues, consider the following tips:

- **Ingredient Substitutions:** If you're having trouble finding certain ingredients, explore alternative options that are readily available in your area. Be creative and experiment with substitutions to achieve similar flavors and textures.
- **Staying Motivated:** Maintaining motivation is key to sticking to your dietary plan. Set realistic goals, celebrate your successes, and seek support from friends, family, or online communities. Remember to focus on the positive changes you're making for your health.
- **Monitoring Progress:** If you're not seeing the desired results, reassess your dietary and lifestyle habits. Are you following the meal plan consistently? Are you incorporating physical activity and managing stress effectively? Making small adjustments and staying committed to your goals can lead to long-term success.

Q: I'm having difficulty finding some of the ingredients listed in the recipes. What should I do? A: If specific ingredients are unavailable, don't fret! Many recipes can be adapted by substituting similar ingredients that are readily available in your area. Feel free to get creative and experiment with alternative ingredients to achieve comparable flavors and textures.

Q: I'm struggling to stick to the meal plan. Any tips for staying motivated? A: Sticking to a new dietary regimen can be challenging, especially in the beginning. To maintain motivation, focus on the positive changes you're making for your health, and celebrate your successes along the way. Set achievable goals, enlist support from friends and family, and reward yourself for staying committed to your health journey.

Q: I'm not seeing the results I expected. What am I doing wrong? A: Achieving health goals takes time and patience, so don't be discouraged if progress is slower than anticipated. Reflect on your dietary and lifestyle habits to identify areas for improvement. Are you following the meal plan consistently? Are you engaging in regular exercise and managing stress effectively? Making small adjustments and staying committed to your goals can lead to long-term success.

These FAQ sections provide detailed responses to common concerns encountered when following the GCA Diet Cookbook. By addressing each question independently, readers can find practical solutions to their specific dietary needs and challenges.

CHAPTER 12

RESOURCES AND FURTHER READING

Exploring additional resources and further reading materials can provide invaluable support and information for managing Giant Cell Arteritis (GCA) and Polymyalgia Rheumatica (PMR). Let's delve into each aspect in comprehensive detail:

1. Recommended Books and Websites:

Books:
Dive deeper into understanding GCA and PMR by exploring a selection of recommended books authored by healthcare professionals, researchers, and individuals with lived experience. These books cover a wide range of topics, including disease management, symptom relief, dietary strategies, and coping mechanisms. Look for titles that provide evidence-based information, practical tips, and personal anecdotes to guide you on your journey with GCA and PMR.

Websites:
Discover authoritative websites dedicated to GCA and PMR, curated by medical institutions, patient advocacy organizations, and research foundations. These websites offer up-to-date information, educational resources, and support networks for individuals affected by these conditions. Explore comprehensive articles, fact sheets, and multimedia resources to deepen your understanding of GCA and PMR. Additionally, engage with online forums, chat rooms, and social media groups to connect with others, share experiences, and access peer support.

2. Support Groups and Communities:

Local Support Groups:
Connect with individuals in your local community who are living with GCA and PMR by joining local support groups. These groups typically meet in-person or virtually to provide a safe space for sharing experiences, exchanging practical advice, and offering emotional support. Participate in group discussions, educational seminars, and social events organized by local support groups to foster meaningful connections and camaraderie.

Online Communities:
Join online support groups and communities dedicated to GCA and PMR to connect with a broader network of individuals from around the world. These virtual communities offer forums, message boards, and social media groups where you can interact with fellow patients, caregivers, and healthcare professionals. Engage in discussions, ask questions, and share resources to gain insights, find encouragement, and build supportive relationships within the GCA and PMR community.

3. Professional Guidance and Consultation:

Rheumatologists and Healthcare Providers:
Consult with rheumatologists, primary care physicians, and other healthcare providers specializing in rheumatology and autoimmune diseases for professional guidance and consultation. Schedule regular appointments to discuss your diagnosis, treatment options, medication management, and symptom relief strategies. Your healthcare team can provide personalized recommendations tailored to your specific needs and health goals.

Registered Dietitians:
Seek guidance from registered dietitians who specialize in autoimmune conditions and inflammatory diseases. A registered dietitian can help you develop a customized dietary plan that supports your overall health and addresses specific nutritional needs related to GCA and PMR. Receive evidence-based nutrition advice, meal planning assistance, and practical tips for incorporating anti-inflammatory foods into your diet.

Physical Therapists and Allied Health Professionals:
Engage with physical therapists and other allied health professionals to explore complementary therapies and rehabilitation strategies for managing symptoms of GCA and PMR. Receive personalized exercise prescriptions, mobility exercises, and pain management techniques to improve joint function, reduce stiffness, and enhance overall quality of life.

By exploring recommended books, websites, support groups, and professional consultation, you can access a wealth of resources and support to empower you on your journey with GCA and PMR.

CONCLUSION

As you conclude your exploration of managing Giant Cell Arteritis (GCA) and Polymyalgia Rheumatica (PMR) through dietary changes and lifestyle adjustments, it's essential to reflect on your journey and look toward the future with optimism and determination. Let's delve into each aspect in comprehensive detail:

1. Embracing Your Healing Journey:

Take a moment to acknowledge the resilience and determination you've demonstrated throughout your healing journey with GCA and Polymyalgia Rheumatica (PMR). Recognize the courage it takes to confront the challenges posed by these conditions and the strength you've shown in adapting to dietary changes and lifestyle adjustments. Embrace a mindset of self-compassion and self-empowerment as you navigate the ups and downs of managing your health.

2. Staying Motivated and Committed:

Maintaining motivation and commitment to your health goals is essential for long-term success. Set realistic expectations for your progress and celebrate each milestone, no matter how small. Cultivate a support network of friends, family, healthcare providers, and fellow patients who can provide encouragement, accountability, and understanding. Remember that setbacks are a natural part of the journey, and resilience lies in your ability to pick yourself up and continue moving forward.

3. Looking Ahead: Long-Term Health and Wellness:

As you look to the future, prioritize your long-term health and wellness by incorporating sustainable dietary habits, lifestyle modifications, and self-care practices into your daily routine. Continue to prioritize anti-inflammatory foods, such as fruits, vegetables, whole grains, and lean proteins, while minimizing processed foods, refined sugars, and unhealthy fats. Engage in regular physical activity, practice stress management techniques such as mindfulness and meditation, and prioritize restorative sleep for optimal well-being.

Stay informed about advancements in treatment options, research findings, and emerging therapies for GCA and PMR by staying connected with healthcare professionals, patient advocacy organizations, and reputable medical resources. Advocate for yourself and actively participate in your healthcare decisions, ensuring that your voice is heard and your needs are met.

As you conclude your journey with the Giant Cell Arteritis Diet Cookbook, remember that you are not alone in your pursuit of health and well-being. By embracing your healing journey, staying motivated and committed, and looking ahead to long-term health and wellness, you can empower yourself to live a vibrant and fulfilling life despite the challenges posed by GCA and PMR.

GLOSSARY OF TERMS

- **Giant Cell Arteritis (GCA):** A chronic inflammatory disease characterized by inflammation of the medium and large arteries, particularly the temporal arteries. Symptoms include severe headaches, scalp tenderness, jaw pain, and vision disturbances.

- **Polymyalgia Rheumatica (PMR):** An inflammatory disorder causing pain and stiffness in the shoulders, neck, hips, and thighs, often accompanied by fatigue, fever, and weight loss.

- **Anti-inflammatory Foods:** Foods rich in antioxidants, vitamins, minerals, and phytonutrients that help reduce inflammation. Examples include fruits, vegetables, whole grains, fatty fish, nuts, seeds, and olive oil.

- **Macronutrients:** Essential nutrients required in large amounts by the body for energy production and growth. Macronutrients include carbohydrates, proteins, and fats.

- **Micronutrients:** Essential nutrients required in smaller amounts for various physiological functions, including vitamins and minerals.

- **Phytonutrients:** Bioactive compounds found in plant foods that have antioxidant and anti-inflammatory properties, helping to protect against chronic diseases.

- **Gluten-Free:** A diet excluding gluten, a protein found in wheat, barley, rye, and related grains, often followed by individuals with celiac disease or gluten sensitivity.

- **Mediterranean Diet:** A dietary pattern emphasizing fruits, vegetables, whole grains, legumes, nuts, seeds, olive oil, fish, and moderate consumption of poultry, eggs, and dairy products.

- **Stress Management Techniques:** Strategies and practices to reduce stress levels and promote relaxation, such as mindfulness meditation, deep breathing exercises, yoga, and tai chi.

- **Nutrient-Dense Foods:** Foods providing a high concentration of essential nutrients relative to their calorie content, including fruits, vegetables, whole grains, lean proteins, and healthy fats.

- **Corticosteroids:** Medications prescribed to reduce inflammation and suppress the immune system in conditions like GCA and PMR.

- **Erythrocyte Sedimentation Rate (ESR):** A blood test measuring the rate at which red blood cells settle in a tube, used to indicate inflammation.

- **C-reactive Protein (CRP):** A substance produced by the liver in response to inflammation, used as a marker of disease activity in GCA and PMR.

- **Temporal Artery Biopsy:** A diagnostic procedure removing a small sample of the temporal artery to confirm inflammation indicative of GCA.

- **Prednisone:** A corticosteroid medication commonly prescribed to manage inflammation and symptoms in GCA and PMR.

- **Methotrexate:** An immunosuppressive medication used as a steroid-sparing agent in GCA and PMR treatment.

- **Fiber:** A type of carbohydrate in plant-based foods that promotes digestive health, regulates blood sugar, and maintains satiety.

- **Omega-3 Fatty Acids:** Essential fatty acids with anti-inflammatory properties found in fatty fish, flaxseeds, chia seeds, and walnuts.

- **Probiotics:** Beneficial bacteria that promote gut health and immune function, found in fermented foods like yogurt, kefir, sauerkraut, and kimchi.

- **Prebiotics:** Non-digestible fibers in foods that fuel probiotics, promoting their growth and activity in the gut.

- **Glucocorticoids:** A class of steroid hormones regulating metabolism, immune function, and inflammation, with synthetic versions used in anti-inflammatory medications.

- **Bone Density:** A measure of bone strength and density, often assessed with a DEXA scan, important for individuals on long-term corticosteroids.

- **Calcium:** A mineral essential for bone health, muscle function, and nerve transmission, crucial for those at risk of bone loss due to corticosteroids.

- **Vitamin D:** A fat-soluble vitamin necessary for calcium absorption and bone health, often supplemented to maintain optimal levels.

- **Inflammatory Markers:** Biomarkers in the blood indicating inflammation, such as ESR and CRP, used to assess disease activity and treatment response.

- **Remission:** A state of significantly reduced or absent disease activity and well-controlled symptoms, a primary treatment goal in GCA and PMR.

- **Relapse:** The recurrence of symptoms after a period of remission, requiring adjustments to medication and management strategies.

- **Flare-up:** A sudden exacerbation of symptoms, characterized by increased pain, stiffness, and inflammation, needing prompt medical attention.

- **Patient Education:** Providing information, resources, and support to individuals with GCA and PMR to enhance their understanding, treatment options, and self-management strategies.

- **Autoimmune Disease:** A condition in which the immune system mistakenly attacks the body's own tissues, leading to inflammation and damage.

- **Dietary Fiber:** Plant-based carbohydrates that cannot be digested, promoting healthy digestion and preventing constipation.

- **Whole Grains:** Grains that contain the entire grain kernel, including the bran, germ, and endosperm, offering more nutrients than refined grains.

- **Lean Proteins:** Protein sources low in fat, such as chicken, turkey, fish, legumes, and tofu, important for muscle maintenance and repair.

- **Healthy Fats:** Fats beneficial for health, including monounsaturated and polyunsaturated fats found in olive oil, avocados, nuts, and fatty fish.

- **Processed Foods:** Foods that have been altered from their natural state through processing, often containing added sugars, unhealthy fats, and preservatives.

- **Refined Sugars:** Sugars extracted and processed from natural sources, often leading to blood sugar spikes and increased inflammation.

- **Oxidative Stress:** An imbalance between free radicals and antioxidants in the body, leading to cellular damage and inflammation.

- **Antioxidants:** Compounds that neutralize free radicals and reduce oxidative stress, found in fruits, vegetables, nuts, and seeds.

- **Immunosuppressants:** Medications that suppress the immune system's activity, used to treat autoimmune conditions by reducing inflammation and preventing tissue damage.

- **Chronic Pain:** Long-term pain persisting beyond the usual course of an illness or injury, common in conditions like GCA and PMR.

- **Joint Stiffness:** A common symptom of PMR, characterized by reduced range of motion and discomfort in the joints, particularly in the morning.

- **Muscle Weakness:** A decrease in muscle strength, often experienced in individuals with PMR due to inflammation and disuse.

- **Fatigue:** A feeling of persistent tiredness and lack of energy, commonly associated with chronic inflammatory conditions like GCA and PMR.

- **Hydration:** The process of maintaining adequate fluid levels in the body, essential for overall health and optimal bodily functions.

- **Elimination Diet:** A diet that removes specific foods or food groups suspected of causing adverse reactions, used to identify food intolerances.

- **Holistic Health:** An approach to health that considers the whole person, including physical, mental, emotional, and social well-being.

- **Complementary Therapies:** Non-mainstream practices used alongside conventional medicine, such as acupuncture, massage, and herbal remedies.

- **Functional Foods:** Foods that provide health benefits beyond basic nutrition, often containing bioactive compounds that promote health and prevent disease.

- **Dietitian:** A healthcare professional specializing in nutrition and dietetics, providing personalized dietary advice and meal planning.

- **Chronic Disease Management:** Ongoing care and support for individuals with long-term conditions to improve quality of life and prevent complications.

www.ingramcontent.com/pod-product-compliance
Lightning Source LLC
Chambersburg PA
CBHW051736170526
45167CB00002B/953